> *And we know that in all things God works for the good of those who love Him, who have been called according to His purpose. (Romans 8:28)*

ALL THINGS WORK FOR GOOD

A Book of Encouragement

for

People with Cancer,

Their Family and Friends

by Gavin Sinclair

With contributions from
Frank Sinclair, Myrle Sinclair, Jennifer Sinclair,
Jennette Sinclair, Mareth Sinclair Gunstream,
Margaret Stauffer, Charlotte Harrington, Vincent Bonaddio,
Robert Barrett, and Christine Hrenya

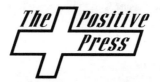

Published by

The Positive Press
P.O. Box 32668
Tucson, AZ 85751-2668

All Scripture quotations are taken from *The Holy Bible, New International Version* (North American Edition), copyright © 1973, 1978, 1984 by the International Bible Society. Used by permission of the Zondervan Publishing House.

10 9 8 7 6 5 4 3 2 1

Publisher's Cataloging in Publication
(Prepared by Quality Books Inc.)

Sinclair, Gavin.
    All things work for good : a book of encouragement for people with cancer, their family and friends / by Gavin Sinclair, with contributions from Frank Sinclair . . .[et al.].
    p. cm.
    Includes bibliographical references and index.
    ISBN 0-9655381-0-9

    1. Sinclair, Gavin. 2. Cancer--Patients--Biography. 3. Cancer--Patients--Family relationships. 4. Cancer--Popular Works. 5. Cancer--Religious aspects. I. Title

RC279.6.C66A3 1997   362.1'96994'0092
                                    QBI96-40717

Contents

ACKNOWLEDGMENTS 7

INTRODUCTION..9

PART I: MY STORY

1. THE DIAGNOSIS..13

2. TREATMENT IN CINCINNATI...19

3. WAITING..29

4. SLOAN-KETTERING 35

5. PARENTHOOD..49

6. THE DARKEST DAYS...57

7. BACK TO WORK..67

8. CONGESTIVE HEART FAILURE...71

9. SPINAL SURGERY 75

10. STROKE! (AND A SCARE)..85

PART II: FROM ANOTHER ANGLE

11. FROM MY WIFE 99

12. FROM MY DAUGHTER..109

13. FROM MY SISTER...111

14. FROM MY FRIENDS 115

PART III: PUTTING IT ALL TOGETHER

15. THE SPIRITUAL LESSONS...125

16. THE MENTAL LESSONS...133

17. THE PHYSICAL LESSONS...139

18. THE FAMILY LESSONS 147

CONCLUDING COMMENTS 153

APPENDIX

HOSPITAL VISITATION 157

ANOTHER STORY..159

FURTHER READING 167

INDEX...169

Acknowledgments

I would like to thank the numerous people who reviewed and made comments on the early copies of the manuscript including my parents, Frank and Myrle Sinclair; my wife Jennifer Sinclair; my sister and brother-in-law, Mareth and Robby Gunstream; my brother-in-law and sister-in-law, Bryan and Amy Doloresco; my mother-in-law, Carolyn Doloresco; and my friends John Cooley, Vinney and Lauri Bonaddio, Ann Rose, Cindy Morrow, Christine Hrenya, Becky DiLorenzo, and special thanks to Diana Lytle, who edited the final manuscript.

A number of people read the manuscript and encouraged me to complete the project including John Davey, Sally Charboneau, Jim and Pam Baygents, Tom and Shannon Peterson, Sunthar Visuvalingam, Chuck and Margaret Stauffer, Bob and Phyllis Hoffman, Tim and Karen Morrison, Diane Stortz, Shirley McKay, Terry and Shirley Morrison, Pete Hrenya, Ross and Maureen Erdis, Marjorie Erdis, and Dharma Singh Khalsa.

Timeline

Early December 1985	Diagnosed with bronchitis in New Jersey
Late December 1985	Diagnosed with cancer in Cincinnati
January-February 1986	Chemotherapy and radiation
March 1986	Home in Flemington, NJ
April 14, 1986	Cancer surgery at Memorial Sloan-Kettering
April 25, 1986	Jennette born
May 30, 1986	Teflon injection to vocal cord
June 1986	Examined in three different hospitals with unknown fever
July 1986	Chemotherapy in Cincinnati
October 1986	Returned to work
April 1988	Moved to Bethlehem, Pennsylvania
August 1988	Congestive heart failure
May 1, 1989	Spinal cord surgery
January 1990	Stopped narcotic drugs, moved to Pittsburgh
September 1990	Stroke
November 1991	Benign tumor
November 1994	Moved to Tucson, Arizona

Introduction

In December 1985, when I was away from home visiting my in-laws, I was diagnosed with terminal cancer. I was 24 years old. My wife was five months pregnant with our first child. I was told I had four months to live.

For the next ten years my world was filled with medical problems and treatments. I had chemotherapy, radiation, and chest surgery to remove the cancer. Then came a stroke, congestive heart failure, spinal surgery, a tracheostomy, vocal cord surgery, physical therapy, speech therapy, a cardiac catheterization, bone scans, MUGA scans, MRIs, and numerous CT scans, all secondary to the original cancer treatment. I started out not even knowing what most of these things were, but in telling my story, I will explain them all.

A person can't go through all these problems without learning something. At my young age, I learned a lot about hospitals, doctors, how friends and family respond and, most importantly, how to face death. This book is the story of my experience with cancer and what I, together with my family and friends, learned from it. If you have gone through a serious illness, I think you will recognize many of the same feelings and experiences. If you are preparing to go through treatments, this book may give you an idea of what to expect.

Over the course of my treatment, I met many people with cancer. It was encouraging to compare "war" stories. I found many people had the same feelings and thoughts when they were first diagnosed, when they had their first chemotherapy or radiation treatment, or when they woke up in the recovery room after surgery. I wish I had heard all those stories before I started my own cancer treatments. There is a lot of comfort in knowing you are not alone.

My family and friends had an equally difficult time during my treatments. Until a loved one has cancer, it is difficult to know how to feel or how to respond to their needs. In this book I have included personal accounts from my friends and family. Reading what they experienced can help others who are helping a friend or family member deal with cancer or another serious illness.

No one has practice facing a serious illness for the first time. We may watch movies or see other people go through it, but it is not the same. When you are the one enduring the illness, it stays with you 24 hours a day, often for month after month or year after year. I had no idea what surviving this long, continuous struggle meant when I was first diagnosed.

Many people have thought about facing death. It's not the same until someone tells you that your time is *now*. Not many people have their lives in order. Most think they have plenty of time. When we find out our days are numbered, we work very hard to straighten out our lives. As I describe in this book, my terminal prognosis forced me to confront some things that I should have faced long before.

As you read this book, remember that I got through all these problems and, at the end, *I was happy I went through it.* I know that's hard to believe, but I hope you'll understand when you reach the end of the book.

Throughout the book I have added thoughts that may be helpful to you. Not everything I say is right for everybody. I hope you will extract the ideas that are useful for your situation, and ignore those things that you may not agree with. Hopefully, I have written some things that will make your experience a little easier.

PART I: MY STORY

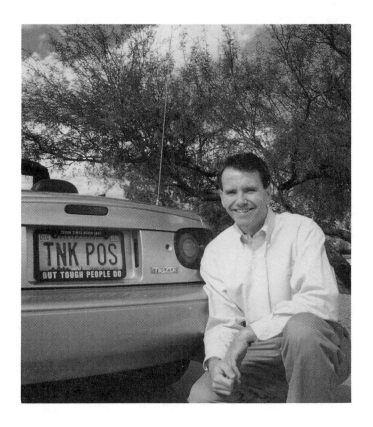

Gavin Sinclair

Chapter 1: The Diagnosis

I felt terrible. I was in a meeting with a chemical sup-
plier discussing whether toluene diisocyanate or methylene
diphenyl isocyanate would become the chemical of choice for
automotive seat cushions. At that point in time (like most other
people in the world), I didn't know and I didn't care. All I
knew was that I felt terrible. I excused myself and made the
two hour drive back to my home in rural New Jersey. As I
crossed the Delaware River, I remember thinking I had never
felt this bad before. I went to my bedroom and collapsed into
bed.

The next day I went to see my family doctor in
Flemington, New Jersey. It was December 1985. The waiting
room was filled with a Christmas tree, Christmas cards, and a
bunch of people that looked as bad as I did. " 'Tis the season,"
I thought, "to pass around germs." I filled out the information
form: Age: 24, Previous health problems: none. After the
typical one hour wait, I went in to see the doctor.

"Bronchitis," he said, after listening to my lungs. He
gave me a prescription for antibiotics. I had the feeling he had

gone through this routine quite often in the past of couple weeks. "Come back in ten days if you are not feeling better," the doctor told me. I went back home to bed.

Following the doctor's instructions to the letter, I was back in ten days showing no improvement. "Sounds the same," the doctor said after putting the cold stethoscope to my chest again. "Let's go another ten days with the antibiotics."

My wife and I were scheduled to visit her family in Cincinnati in about five days. My wife Jennifer was a graduate student in Chemical Engineering at Princeton, and she didn't get to see her mother very often. Jennifer was also five months pregnant with our first child, so she was especially eager to go to Cincinnati. On the appointed day our next-door-neighbors, George and Charlotte Riley, loaded me into the back seat of our car to go to the airport. We drove to the airport and flew to Cincinnati.

My mother-in-law was a receptionist for a doctor in Cincinnati, and she worked me into the doctor's schedule the next day. I went to the office (no waiting this time, thanks to my "connections"), and Dr. Richards went through the usual routine. He calmly told me to go to the hospital for an x-ray. I didn't know it at the time, but he suspected problems. He told my mother-in-law later that my breathing sounds were poor.

I went for the x-ray, my first one ever. Even though I still felt terrible, I was fascinated by the hospital procedures, probably the result of watching too much *Medical Center* and *Marcus Welby, M.D.* as a kid. My mother-in-law told me the results of the x-ray that evening. She was very calm and pro-fessional. She had the foresight to tell my wife earlier that day.

"The x-ray shows a large mass in the chest," she told me. "The doctors think it is probably a lymphoma." At that point, I didn't make the connection to cancer. Lymphoma sounds less serious, like an overactive gland or something. I wasn't overly concerned.

The next day I went back to see Dr. Richards. My father came over from Indianapolis to go with me. The doctor sounded serious, and he wanted me admitted into the hospital right away. I still wasn't worried. "It won't take me long to get over this," I thought. I had things to do at home.

After the appointment, my father called my sister in Colorado to tell her the news. Before he could finish the story, he broke into tears and had to hang up. I thought he was taking things too seriously, and I immediately called my sister back so she wouldn't worry. "It's no big deal," I told her. "It's not like I'm going to die or anything." Many times in the coming months I would think about that conversation. It turned out death was more likely than life.

I was admitted to Providence Hospital later that day. It was all very interesting to me. I had never been in the hospital before. I was introduced to Dr. Morgan, the oncologist who was handling my case. I didn't even know what an oncologist was. I was 24 years old. I had never needed to know what an oncologist was. I looked it up and learned that an oncologist was a doctor who specialized in the treatment of cancer. "Oh, yeah," I thought. "I guess I do have something that could be classified as cancer. But not *cancer*."

One of the first things they did was a needle biopsy. Although a lymphoma would be the typical type of cancer to strike someone of my age, they needed to get a sample of tissue from the tumor to make sure. I was given a shot that made me groggy, and then I was wheeled to the operating room. When I got there, they started prepping me for the procedure by swabbing the right side of my chest. "Excuse me," I said, "but shouldn't you be swabbing the other side?"

The nurse looked up at the x-ray and said, "Oh yeah. I guess you're right." The combination of drugs and my general attitude made this a very humorous experience. I repeated this story to all my friends. I still wasn't taking things too seriously. My attitude would quickly change.

When I was visiting my parents over Thanksgiving vacation just one month earlier, I had a long conversation with my father. I told him I thought that life had been too easy for me. In high school I was a class officer, president of the science and writing clubs, captain of the golf team, and a top student. I was the youngest member of the Indianapolis Symphonic Choir and sang in Carnegie Hall and Kennedy Center. In college I graduated with double degrees in Chemical Engineering and Industrial Management in only four years, and still found the time to marry a beautiful and intelligent classmate ranked first in our class. I was hired by a major corporation at a good salary, and my wife enrolled in graduate school at Princeton University. We bought a colonial house in a rural area of New Jersey. We were expecting our first child. I seemed to have a pretty good life.

In fact, I felt my life had been too good. In the conversation with my father, I suggested that most opportunities seem to come from adversity. A war creates the opportunity to become a hero. Being fired from a safe, secure job offers the motivation to start a new business. My life was running along very smoothly, and I didn't see how I would ever get the opportunity to accomplish anything really important with my life.

They say you should be careful what you wish for, because your wish might just come true. I was looking for adversity, and I found it.

The hospital in Cincinnati could not make a definite identification of the tumor, so they sent the biopsy sample to the Cleveland Clinic. The laboratory in Cleveland took a long time analyzing the tissue samples from the biopsy. So long, in fact, that Dr. Morgan started radiation and chemotherapy before the final result was in. They finally reached a conclusion. Dr. Morgan came into my hospital room and wrote on a piece of paper, *Malignant fibrous hystiocytoma (sarcoma).* He told me this is a rare type of cancer to show up in the chest, especially in a person my age. Dr. Morgan had only seen one case like mine in the past six years. "How serious is it?" I asked.

"You probably have four months. Maybe up to two years if you respond well to treatment," Dr. Morgan answered. I remember sneaking into the nurse's closet that night to read my chart. Commenting on the biopsy report from the Cleveland Clinic, Dr. Morgan had written, "Worst diagnosis possible."

Four months to live. Reality finally set in. It didn't seem like a little gland problem anymore.

People react differently when they are told they have four months to live. Some don't believe it. Some get angry. Some want to be comforted by others. I just wanted to be left alone.

"Four months to live is a long way from bronchitis," I thought, remembering my family doctor's diagnosis. My first reaction was to be angry with my family doctor. "A simple x-ray would have shown the tumor," I thought.

In retrospect, I was very fortunate that the first doctor made the wrong diagnosis. First, it showed me that doctors can be wrong. If you've never been sick before, the tendency is to believe whatever the doctor tells you. As my story unfolds, you'll see this is a bad assumption. The misdiagnosis taught me very early in the process *that I had to be responsible for my own care.* Second, the medical facilities in Cincinnati were much better than the ones where I was living in New Jersey. And since I was being treated in Cincinnati, my family was also nearby (my parents in Indianapolis, Jennifer's family in Cincinnati). Without the support and help from our parents, my cancer treatments would have been much more difficult.

Next, I started to think about death. I had never given much thought to death before. I was 24 years old. Death was on my mind a lot for the next few days. I decided that to face death I had to confront two questions. The first question was whether I was happy with what I had accomplished on earth. I had a great deal of trouble with this one. I was always preparing for the future. I never gave much thought to what I was accomplishing *now*. I was sorry that (apparently) I had learned this lesson too late.

Second, I needed to know where I was going when I died. I'm sure death is very scary to people who have no beliefs. I had no problems with this one. I am a Christian, and I knew I was going to heaven.

A friend of mine, John Davey, once gave a sermon about turning "head nods into heart nods." If you ask a Christian if they are going to heaven when they die, they will dutifully nod their head "yes." After all, they learned this in Sunday school. But a head nod is different from a heart nod. If you believe in your heart that you are going to heaven, there is no fear in death. Heaven is a better place than earth. If you believe in your heart that you are going to heaven when you die, much of the stress of your illness goes away. When the stress is gone, you are better able to fight the disease.

The natural question for most people is "What about my family?" I had parents, a wife, and an unborn baby. Even if I'm happy in heaven, what about them? The apostle Paul wrote in Romans, "And we know that in all things God works for the good of those who love Him, who have been called according to His purpose." (Romans 8:28) This became my cornerstone through many years of trials. If you truly believe that all things work for good, you can be confident that God will take care of your family. I realized that my responsibility was to love God and seek His will, and He would take care of the rest.

Chapter 2: Treatment in Cincinnati

I had three principal doctors in the hospital. Dr. Morgan was my primary doctor and the one who administered chemotherapy. The second doctor was a radiation oncologist. He was the doctor who decided how radiation could be used to help cure the cancer. The third doctor was a surgeon. Chemotherapy, radiation, and surgery are three conventional treatments for cancer. I am not a medical doctor, but let me give you the layperson's explanation of these three types of treatments.

Chemotherapy is where chemicals are injected into the patient to kill the cancer cells throughout the body. Different chemicals are effective against different kinds of tumors. The chemotherapy can also do damage to normal cells, especially fast-growing cells like those lining the stomach walls and hair follicles. (This is the reason why nausea and hair loss can be side effects of chemotherapy.) There are usually multiple treatments, often on a weekly or monthly basis.

Radiation is a treatment that is aimed directly at the tumor. This treatment is specific to the region of the tumor. If the cancer is fairly localized, radiation can be a very effective treatment. Radiation also involves multiple treatments, often daily treatments for a few months.

Surgery, of course, is simply going in and cutting out the tumor. Surgery is not always an option if the tumor is in a difficult location.

The chemotherapy and radiation doctors both established plans for my treatment. The surgeon decided to pass. "The tumor is growing into the heart, and it would be too dangerous to try to cut the tumor out," he told me. "Maybe if the chemotherapy or radiation shrinks the tumor we could try, but I doubt it. The tumor is basically inoperable."

The surgeon did do a tracheostomy on me so I could lie flat to get the radiation treatments. A tracheostomy is an operation where they put a tube into your throat, and then you breathe through the tube. Before the tracheostomy I was unable to lie flat because my breathing was being cut off by the tumor pushing against the airway. Once the tracheostomy was done, I began radiation and chemotherapy.

After a few weeks of chemotherapy and radiation, I came to an important conclusion: *The only thing worse than dying of cancer is being treated for it.*

I was not a good chemotherapy patient. My first treatment was New Year's Eve. I got the treatment late in the evening, with the theory that I would sleep through the worst of it. Wrong. I was throwing up every fifteen minutes. One of the nurses came in after midnight and said, "I just left a party where people were throwing up just like you." Not a very comforting thought, to tell you the truth. I threw up (or at least went through the motions) for three straight days. I felt like a wet dishrag.

Even though I got very sick from the chemotherapy, I never lost all of my hair. Many patients have a hard time dealing with going bald, and bandannas and wigs are good options. I think Dr. Morgan was a little disappointed that I didn't go bald, because hair loss at least shows the chemotherapy is doing something.

I would have dealt better with chemotherapy if I had been mentally prepared. I started my first treatment exactly three days after learning what an "oncologist" was. All I knew was people told me that chemotherapy would make me feel very sick. That's what I expected, and that's what I got. As I started reading books about cancer, I began to learn that the "mind-body connection" is very strong. If you *think* chemotherapy will make you sick, it *will* make you sick. Being a logical engineer, I was skeptical that the mind could cause physical illness. Then I read that 30% of chemotherapy patients throw up *on the way* to treatment. That's a pretty telling statistic, and it made a believer out of me.

My wife hates tea. The reason she hates tea is because her father always gave her tea when she was sick, so she associates tea with being sick. This is another example of the mind-body connection.

You can make the mind-body connection work for you by telling yourself that chemotherapy is a treatment to help you, and many people have chemotherapy with hardly any side effects. In fact, anti-nausea drugs get better every year, so there is no reason to assume that chemotherapy will make you sick. I wish I had known that before I started chemotherapy.

I was ready for radiation, though. The first thing the radiation oncologist did was carefully measure out the precise area to receive radiation. He wanted to focus the radiation carefully to get the maximum effect on the tumor while minimizing the effect on normal cells. It took about four hours for the doctor to take x-rays, make a mold for the area that was to receive radiation, and mark my body with indelible "X's" used to aim the radiation. At the end of the layout session, I looked like a human "tic-tac-toe" board. Once the area was carefully measured, the treatments were very easy. I went in once a day and lay down on the treatment table. The technician aimed a beam of light at my target "X," turned on the radiation machine for a few minutes, and I was done.

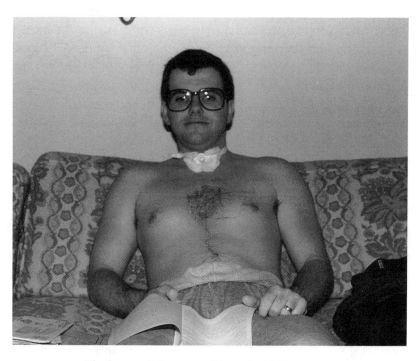

The human "tic-tac-toe" board with his trach

I decided that radiation was my friend. Whenever I lay on the table getting the treatment, I visualized Jesus leading a team of "Pac-man" invaders eating up the tumor. For those who don't remember the early video games, Pac-man was a game where these circle-shaped creatures with big mouths would gobble up "food" and other creatures. It sounds ridiculous, but I think visualizing my Pac-man invaders was important to help get my mind fighting the disease and to maintain a positive attitude. I never had any problems with radiation, and my mental efforts gave me an outlet to do something that could contribute to my situation rather than just feeling helpless.

Some Christians I have talked to don't believe that visualization is right. I'm not sure why, but they seem to conjure up thoughts of voodoo and black magic. Visualization is really just concentrating on a certain thought. As with anything, if you concentrate on the wrong thing, that can be harmful. But if you concentrate on a Christ-centered thought (like I did with Jesus leading the charge of my Pac-man invaders), I do not believe there is a problem.

Others oppose visualization because they don't see how it can help. But as Dr. Morgan said to me when I told him what I was doing, "It can't hurt." The fact is, studies have shown that people who use visualization have a better cure rate. A good book on visualization is *Getting Well Again* (see *Further Reading* in the Appendix).

Unfortunately, the x-rays did not show the progress my "Pac-man" warriors were making. Periodic x-rays showed the tumor was not shrinking. Every night my two-year-old nephew in Boulder, Colorado would pray, "Tumor shrink. Gavin get better." So far, his prayers did not seem to be answered.

Periodically, the doctors would order a CT (computerized tomography) scan to get a better idea of the size of the tumor. A CT scan gives the doctor a three-dimensional view by taking a series of cross-sectional x-rays. To get a CT scan, you lie on a table and the table moves your body through a piece of equipment resembling a giant donut. Usually the technician injects you with a contrast solution to make the images more clear. It is a very strange sensation for the first couple of minutes after they inject the contrast solution. You can actually feel a "hot wave" passing through your body, like a heating pad that expands from your arm and gradually covers your entire body. The first time I had this test, I thought I was having an adverse reaction to the injection, but it is actually all very normal. Once I did have a reaction to the CT scan dye which caused hives. I took one antihistamine pill and I was fine.

Meanwhile, through all these early treatments, I could not talk. When they do a tracheostomy, you can't talk because the air never gets up to your mouth. Someone got me one of those kid's erasable slates to write messages on. I could have reacted to this with frustration, but I quickly learned that humor was a better response to all of my trials. My sister got caught up in the humor mood when she wrote a "hospital question-naire" for me to fill out.

Besides humor serving as a good substitute for frustra-tion during times of trials, laughter is also very good physi-cally. When you laugh, the body releases endorphins, which are natural painkillers. Laughter also activates the immune system and improves blood circulation. There is a well-know story of Norman Cousins employing laughter as the best medicine. He tells his story in *Anatomy of an Illness*.

I was in the hospital for a little over two weeks. During that time I had many discussions with my main daytime nurse, Mary, using my slate or a battery-powered amplifier that I held against my throat (and made me sound like a robot). A good nurse can make all the difference. She was very kind and helped me understand all the hospital procedures. She was also very nice to my wife and parents.

It wasn't until I was in the hospital for over a week that one of the other nurses told me Mary's husband had died three weeks earlier, leaving her alone with a twelve-year-old son. All the time she had devoted to helping me with my problems, I had no idea of what she had going on in her life at the time. After learning about the death of her husband, I viewed Mary in a new light, amazed at how she was helping other people while coping with her loss. My experience with Mary also made me realize that people were evaluating me in the same way. People were watching me to see how I would handle a serious illness with a terminal prognosis.

Mareth's Hospital Questionnaire

When you come to visit me, I would like you to:
_____ Talk about everything, rapid-style conversation
_____ Talk only when "slated" to (refers to writing
     on my slate)
_____ Talk if I have something interesting to say

I would like visitors:
_____ One at a time
_____ Two at a time
_____ As many as can fit in the room
_____ Sick of visitors

I would like to talk about _____ the most:
_____ Money, financial-related topics
_____ Chemical engineering, and how it relates to all
     aspects of life

I prefer your visit to last:
_____ Under two minutes
_____ Two – thirty minutes
_____ Pajama party
_____ During sporting events
_____ Not during sporting events
     (More than one box can be checked)

When you come, would you please bring:
_____ Cash, check, or money order
_____ Flowers or plant
_____ Chicken soup

When you pray, please pray for:
_____ My tumor
_____ My "trach" (my tracheostomy operation)
_____ A computerized slate
_____ A food grinder

I had many visitors, calls and cards from people during my two weeks in the hospital. When you are fighting an illness, people study you to decide how you are handling things. Everything you do is interpreted in terms of your illness. Here are the typical comments you hear around a hospital:

"He's having a bad day. He's in a lot of pain."

"It's a good day. She got a good report from the doctor."

"I don't think he can take much more. I think he's giving up."

"I don't know how she does it. She is in constant pain, she has tubes stuck into her arm, and yet she was helping the patient across the hall this morning."

While I was in the hospital, I decided there was no better chance to be a good witness to my Christian faith than during a severe illness. First, people expect you to react badly. When you react positively in spite of all your problems, it makes a powerful statement. Doctors and nurses are especially perceptive to this. They see many patients, and they can tell which ones are "different" and respond to their illness with courage. When they start to understand that the common factor is Christian faith, it makes a strong statement.

During a hospital stay, you will also come in contact with many people who are doing a lot of soul-searching. Patients facing death, as well as their family members, are all trying to come to grips with their own mortality. You can give them the answers they are seeking.

The reverse is also true. If you are a Christian openly afraid of dying, people will look at this and wonder why your religion does not give you the confidence of an afterlife. If you are a Christian and constantly complain, people will wonder why your Christianity does not provide you with a way to handle hardship.

After I was released from the hospital, I continued to go in for radiation every day as an outpatient. My weight had fallen from 155 pounds to about 120 pounds, mainly because of my reaction to chemotherapy. I considered starting a company to compete with Weight Watchers and offer "Chemotabs" containing Adriamycin and Cisplatin, two of my chemotherapy drugs.

My five-week period of outpatient radiation gave me a good chance to recover. Steroids are often prescribed for radiation patients to help build you up. In my case, I took Prednisone. After three weeks on Prednisone, I was back up to 155 pounds. I ate everything in sight. I was ready to eat the tires off my car. I was also able to do some work, mailing in reports and memos to my boss.

I went back on my diet with one last outpatient chemotherapy treatment on Valentine's Day. Thankfully, nobody offered me any candy. I finished the famous report on the future of the automotive seating market (remember that critical question of toluene diisocyanate or methylene diphenyl isocyanate) at the cancer center before I started throwing up.

My outpatient treatments were completed in mid-February 1986. Jennifer and I were very comfortable living in Cincinnati, but you can only live with your in-laws for so long. After two months away from home, I was eager to get back.

Fortunately, the move seemed good for my medical condition as well. Moving back to New Jersey meant I would only be a two hour drive away from Memorial Sloan-Kettering Cancer Center in New York, generally regarded as one of the finest cancer hospitals in the world. Dr. Morgan referred me to a doctor who specialized in sarcomas. The Cincinnati doctors had done all they could for me. The tumor was still as big as ever in the x-ray. The question was whether the tumor was now dead tissue, or whether there were some live cancer cells left.

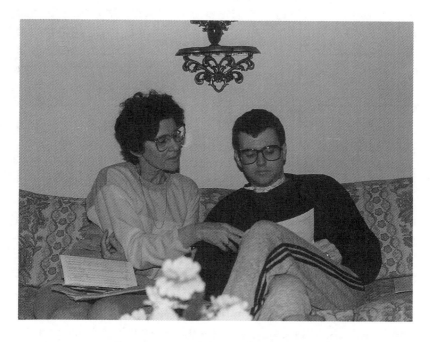

Even cancer patients need to pay taxes.
Here my mother and I try to figure out the latest tax rules.
This picture was taken when I still had my trach.

Chapter 3: Waiting

I spent the month of March 1986 waiting to see what the doctors at Memorial Sloan-Kettering were going to do. All of my records had been sent from Cincinnati, and I was in no hurry for them to tell me I needed more chemotherapy. Jennifer was getting bigger and bigger (as in pregnant), with the baby due in late April. I still had a football-sized tumor in my chest. I didn't know when the tumor might grow a little too close to my heart, or press against a vital nerve, and take my life away.

I wondered if I would still be alive to see the baby born, to find out whether the baby was a boy or a girl, and whether the baby would ever get to know me. One day I sat down at my computer and wrote a letter to my unborn baby. Here is the introduction:

March 13, 1986

Dear _____

    I'm writing this rather long letter in case I'm not around to tell you the stories it contains. I'm sorry I can't be with you, but at least you can read whatever interesting stories I can think of. Almost like an edited version of a father–all the good stories with the boring stuff cut out.

    I guess I feel like I cheated you. No one should have to grow up without a father. Unfortunately, it wasn't my idea to leave this earth a little early. Hopefully this letter will help make up for some of the things you've missed.

    I was cheated too. I was very fortunate in my life, and most things turned out well. But I never got to know you, and that disappointment outweighs all the good things combined.

        Love,

        Dad

The letter was very long. I wrote about my favorite books and movies. I wrote about my experiences in high school and college. I wanted my child to know his father, even if he or she could never meet me. But I kept coming back to the first line: "Dear _____." I didn't even know what my child's name would be. I didn't know if I would have a son or a daughter.

When I was first diagnosed with cancer and given four months to live, one of my friends had done some mental math and said, "That means you are going to die at about the same time the baby is born." Writing the letter just reinforced that thought in my mind.

As I wrote the letter, I started to believe that I would not die. My wife was going to have a baby, and I had responsibilities. Although I was still ready to accept whatever God's will might be, I started to believe that God wanted me to live. My baby needed me, and I hoped my story might help other people.

Until I sat down to write the letter to my unborn child, I was not sure what God's plan was for me. I was ready to accept death, if that's what He wanted. Winning the fight is not to get well, but to do the will of God. It is not always God's will to heal a person. Look at the case of Paul in II Corinthians 12. Paul prayed three times for God to remove his affliction. All three times God said "No." Paul's affliction was left by God to remind Paul to remain humble. Paul accepted God's will.

I couldn't help but wonder at times, "Why did this happen to me? Why did I get sick? What did I do?" Some people torment themselves for hours over these questions. The book of Job is a famous story of the "why" question. After pages and pages of evaluation by Job's friends, they still didn't have a clue.

Early on I decided I probably wasn't going to figure out *why*. Instead, I decided to look at my life and do the one thing I could do: resolve anything that was wrong. The Gospel of John, Chapter 5, tells the story of the leper who waited by the pool watching for the stirring of the waters, hoping that he could be the first to reach the water to be healed. Jesus came along and healed him, and told him not to sin any more or something worse might happen to him. I'm not sure if this means that a person's sin can cause illness, but when you have terminal cancer, the thought certainly crosses your mind. Whether sin caused my illness or not, I knew the right thing to do was to confess my sins and try not to sin anymore.

It wasn't too difficult for me to come up with a list of sins. Unrepented sin was a big one. Not forgiving other people was another. After doing my best to correct these problems and then asking God for forgiveness, I moved on. I didn't know if my sins were the reason for my sickness, but by asking for forgiveness, I knew that I had done everything that I could on this subject. From a strictly physical standpoint, the stress caused by not having your life in order can easily lead to sickness. Stress inhibits your immune system and makes your body more vulnerable to sickness.

Another possibility was my sickness would be used to glorify God. The Gospel of John, Chapter 9 tells about when the disciples brought a blind man to Jesus and asked whether the blindness was caused by the man's sin or his parents' sin. Jesus replied it was neither, but instead he was born blind so the works of God could be displayed in him.

I don't think you can ever know for sure the reason *why*. *"Why"* is not really the question. *"How am I going to respond?"* is the real question. I think we need to do what we can in terms of correcting our lives and then move on.

My dedication to live motivated me to improve my physical condition. I started regular exercise, walking laps around our housing development. I read books about nutrition and tried to follow the proper guidelines, including a detour into "yin" and "yang" foods, which really just says to eat a balanced diet including low-fat, high-fiber foods, especially vegetables and fruits. Ever since chemotherapy, the thought of red meat made me positively ill, so that helped with the diet too.

I also took this break from medical treatment to get my everyday life in order. I was only getting 60% of my salary through disability. This is another source of stress that sick people don't need. I found if you write a letter to your creditors explaining your situation and then make an effort to pay something on each bill every month, the bill collectors tend to leave you alone. This is another case where you should do what you can to improve the situation and then trust God for the rest.

I remember once when a friend from work came to visit me at my home—a very *big* friend. I had put out a bowl of potato chips, which he devoured in no time flat. After he finished, he was kind enough to ask if I was doing okay financially. I told him I was doing fine until he ate the only food I had left for dinner.

The month in New Jersey while waiting for the doctors at Sloan-Kettering to decide on a treatment plan was the last time I was to feel reasonably good for the next five years. That's a pretty amazing statement given what I had already been through in Cincinnati for two months. Once the roller coaster started at Sloan-Kettering, I barely had the strength to survive. I'm glad I had this time to reflect, because I reinforced some thoughts that I needed to remember during the tough times.

I already said my greatest comfort was knowing that *all things would work for good*. Without that promise, I never would have made it. The other thing I concentrated on was to try to stay thankful for what I did have. Maybe you think you have it bad, but you can always find someone worse off. Be thankful you don't have what they have. Even if you've lost one arm to cancer, there is certainly someone else who has lost two arms. Without being gruesome, the point is to be thankful for what you have.

Whenever I started feeling sorry for myself in the hospital, I would visit the children's ward. These children were struck down before they even got started in life. I never felt bad for myself after I saw what these children were going through. My feelings of thankfulness were multiplied even more when I paid attention to how the parents of these children were suffering.

My other way of trying to remember to be thankful was to imagine being a prisoner of war. Even with all the suffering I went through in the hospital, at least I knew the doctors and nurses were doing all they could to make me comfortable. Imagine if the doctors and nurses were actually giving me pain through torture. I had family and friends to help me through. POWs have no one. I quickly became thankful for my situation.

Was this a mental game? In part, I suppose it was. Did it help me to remember to be thankful, even though that was difficult at times? Absolutely. It is very easy to lose perspective during a serious illness. I think we need to use every technique possible to help us remember what is important and maintain the proper perspective.

When I was in the hospital, I met a man who had cancer of the tongue. The doctors had cut out his tongue, and he couldn't talk. Even with my terrible prognosis, I never would have traded places with him. He probably wouldn't have wanted to trade places with me either. A person rises to the challenge they are given. God never gives you more than you can handle. Be thankful for what you have.

Chapter 4: Sloan-Kettering

I finally got a call in late March 1986 from Sloan-Kettering. I made an appointment to see one of their oncologists that specialized in soft cell sarcomas. I was immediately encouraged that Sloan-Kettering had doctors who specialized in my specific cancer.

The drive from Flemington, New Jersey to Memorial Sloan-Kettering in New York City took me across Interstate 78, through the Holland Tunnel and Chinatown, and up the East Side past the UN Building. My very pregnant wife and my parents were with me.

We entered Sloan-Kettering and went up an escalator into a beautiful reception area. We were given directions to the oncologist offices and made the long walk to the other side of the center. Along the hallways were pictures of the different cancer research programs taking place at Sloan-Kettering. Now this inspired confidence. I knew I was in the best cancer center in the world.

We ended up in the largest waiting room I had ever seen, completely packed with people. I guess if you are the best cancer center in the world, you also end up being very popular. The receptionist told me they were two hours behind schedule, and it was only 10 a.m.

After waiting several hours, the nurse finally called my name. She took my vital signs, and then Jennifer and I waited in one of the clinic rooms. Shortly thereafter, a resident came in, asked about my medical history, and did an exam. We waited another half hour, and finally the main doctor came in. He had spoken with the resident, and he asked me a few follow-up questions. Then he told me his plan.

"It doesn't look like your chemotherapy was very strong," he told me. "We are going to hit you a lot harder." Harder? I wanted to tell him the easy stuff almost killed me. "I'm going to order a stress test to see if your heart can take the chemotherapy I have planned," the oncologist told me. Another comment that gave me great comfort. "I'll show your x-rays to the surgeons, but I doubt if they will do anything. The only option is chemotherapy." He left to move on to his next patient. I started out the day pretty confident, but ended it completely terrified!

The next day I went back to Sloan-Kettering for my stress test. Another two hours of driving back and forth, fighting the New York City traffic. I had to sign a release form that said they took all the precautions possible, but if I had a heart attack and died during the test, it wasn't their fault. They also informed me a cardiologist was standing by just in case. I had enough stress before I even started the test. The test turned out to be pretty easy. I just had to ride a stationary bike, and they recorded my heart performance.

A week later I had my follow-up appointment with the oncologist. Jennifer said we were going to the "bus station hospital," which was a pretty accurate description of the doctor's waiting room. The doctor was two hours behind again. I was getting the feeling that the "two hour" estimate was standard protocol. I was ushered in to see the resident, who

Jennifer had renamed "the warm-up doctor." The resident asked me why I was there. I told him I thought I was there because the doctor had ordered a stress test to see if my heart could take the chemotherapy. Nothing like getting that personal touch. The resident leafed though my file and left.

A few minutes later, the "real" doctor came in. "How are you feeling?" he asked. Fine, I told him. "Are you having any breathing problems?" No. "Can you walk up stairs?" Yes. "Well, I can't seem to find the results of your stress test, but it sounds like you are okay. I'll go ahead and order the chemotherapy."

I couldn't believe it. I took all the time to go to New York for the stress test, my insurance company was nice enough to pay $750 for the procedure, and now this guy was going ahead with the chemotherapy without even finding the stress test results?

Wanting to stall, I asked if he had shown my x-ray to the surgeon. "No," he said. "But I don't think they will want to operate." I asked if he could get the evaluation from the surgeon before he started the chemotherapy. "Okay," he said, and left.

The future looked pretty bad. This guy said my previous chemotherapy was nothing, and he was going to give me a "strong" treatment. They lost my stress test results, but since I told him I could walk up stairs, he figured I would be able to handle the chemotherapy. And this was all happening at the best cancer center in the world.

A couple of days later I got a call back, this time from the oncologist himself. "I can't believe it, but the surgeon said he would do it. I'll hold off on the chemotherapy for now. We can do more chemotherapy after the surgery." I was so afraid of getting this guy's chemotherapy, I was actually happy that some surgeon decided to try what everyone else said was an impossible task.

Jennifer and I went back to Sloan-Kettering to meet the surgeon on Tuesday, April 8. This time there was no waiting and no warm-up doctor. We were taken immediately to see the surgeon, Dr. Barnes. After a short examination, Dr. Barnes said he would do his best to remove the tumor, but there was a good chance that I could die on the table. He said he would probably have to remove the left lung and one rib. After reflecting for a few seconds, I said to go ahead.

Dr. Barnes told me he could do the surgery on the following Monday, six days away. I don't know what I was expecting, but I didn't think it would happen that quickly. "There is nothing to gain from waiting," Dr. Barnes told me. "The tumor could be growing, and you are forming more and more scar tissue from the radiation. The sooner we do the operation, the better."

I was admitted to Memorial Sloan-Kettering Hospital on Thursday, two days after the appointment with Dr. Barnes. Everything was very well planned and efficient. "I guess if they're going to cut you up, they take things seriously," I told my friends.

The medical support functions at Sloan-Kettering were really outstanding. After I started getting chemotherapy in Cincinnati, nurses had a hard time drawing blood from me. At Sloan-Kettering, they had an Asian gentleman that must have been recruited from an acupuncture clinic. The first thing he did was a Kung Fu routine on my arm. Then when the vein was sticking up really well–w*ham!*–he would stick me with the needle. He always got his vein. I really missed him when staying in other hospitals later, because sometimes it's the little things like drawing blood that cause a lot of pain and frustration.

That weekend I watched Jack Nicklaus, my favorite golfer, win the Masters at age 46 when everyone said it was impossible for him to win. I thought that was a good sign.

Jack Nicklaus

April 28, 1986

Dear Gavin:

    I heard that you haven't been feeling too well lately and just thought I'd drop you a note to let you know I'm thinking about you. You've got a lot of friends pulling for you, and I hope you'll consider me one of them. Just remember this: if I can win the Masters for my sixth time at age 46, then nothing's impossible!

    I hope you're back on your feet again very soon.

Best regards,

Mr. Gavin Sinclair
58 Wellington Avenue
Flemington, New Jersey 08822

/mk

11760 U. S. Highway #1, North Palm Beach, Florida 33408

Letter from Jack Nicklaus

The nurses woke me up at 5 a.m. on Monday to prep me for surgery. Now things were really efficient. I took back all the bad things I had thought about Sloan-Kettering. I saw Jennifer and my parents before they wheeled me to the operating room. I told my father to page Dr. Gannon (that means something to people who grew up watching *Medical Center*).

Waiting in the pre-op room, I wondered if this was the end. I could literally be dead by the end of the day. Still, I felt very peaceful (aided, I'm sure, by the pre-op drugs). I remember looking at the other patients in the pre-op room and wondering what they were thinking.

I was wheeled into the operating room at the appointed time, and I was amazed by how bright it was. Dr. Barnes asked if I was okay, I nodded yes, and one or two seconds later everything went blank.

The next thing I remember was seeing a bright light at the end of a tunnel. I vaguely remembered this was what people who came back from the dead said they saw during the time they were "dead." I was trying to figure out if I was dead or alive.

I slowly started to remember what had happened, that I was in the hospital for surgery. Then I heard the voice of a nurse telling me to wake up, and I felt her taking out my breathing tube. Gradually I started to recall more and realized that I was in the recovery room. Everything still seemed very slow and peaceful. I remember trying to feel my chest to figure out if they had taken out a rib. Eventually Dr. Barnes came and told me the surgery had gone well, and he would see me the next morning.

The next morning I was back in my room feeling great. I was sitting up in bed talking to my friends at work. Dr. Barnes came in, and I told him this surgery was nothing. "Wait a day and see if you still feel that way," he told me.

Dr. Barnes told me the surgery had taken over six hours, and he had removed the tumor along with the upper lobe of the left lung and the sac around the heart. He had implanted 106 radioactive seeds in my chest to kill any remaining cancer cells. The pathology of the tumor showed that 98% of the tumor was necrotic, or dead. Apparently the radiation and "weak" chemotherapy had done a pretty good job.

During the surgery Dr. Barnes had to sacrifice (cut) the nerve that went to my left diaphragm and the nerve that went to one of my vocal cords because these nerves were tangled up in the tumor. The diaphragm is what moves the lung, so the half lung remaining on the left side was pretty much useless. One of the two vocal cords was now paralyzed in place, so the vocal cords could not come together firmly. As a result, I could only whisper. Dr. Barnes said a throat surgeon could inject Teflon into the paralyzed vocal cord, swelling it and allowing the two vocal cords to meet together, giving me a fairly normal voice. I was glad I didn't have to go back to the magic slate again.

Sure enough, just as Dr. Barnes had predicted, the next day I was in agony. I had an incision down the middle of my chest, and then another one that ran sideways across my left chest. The incisions were stitched and taped. The surgeon had to split apart my chest bone to open my chest during the operation, and this bone was now wired together. The wires protruded through the chest enough that you could feel them. The worst part was the nurses made me cough at regular times to clear out my lungs. I felt like my chest was going to burst open. The nurses would even wake me up during the night and make me cough.

Everyone on my floor was a chest patient, so we were all going through the same routine. After surgery the doctors implanted drainage tubes in the lower part of the chest. These tubes came out of the chest and were connected to a bottle that was mounted on wheels. Everyone on the floor would walk around dragging these little drainage carts with tubes sticking into their chests.

After most major surgeries, the doctors do their best to get you up and around as soon as possible—usually long before the patient feels that he or she is ready. But getting up and around helps to speed the body's recovery. I found this to be an ideal example of the importance of setting goals.

I decided I would get up and sit in a chair the first day after surgery. The second day I decided to walk to the door and back. The third day I decided to walk to the end of the hall and back. These seem like simple goals, but in my condition, every step felt like running a marathon. Robert Schuller, the minister with the television broadcast *The Hour of Power*, has an expression, "Inch by inch, everything's a cinch." I tried to keep these words in mind.

If I had started from the perspective that getting up and sitting in a chair was not very meaningful, I would have missed the chance to start making progress. Failing to take the first step would have prevented the second step, and so forth. If you get in the habit of making positive progress toward recovery every day, it gives you a feeling of success that breeds further success.

I never understand why people automatically put on gowns or pajamas when they go into the hospital. I guess it is easier for the doctors and nurses, but usually the only people wearing pajamas in the middle of the day are sick people. The surest way to make yourself feel sick is to put on pajamas in the middle of the day. I wore sweat pants to make me feel like I was working out.

Surgery requires all the emotional strength that you can summon. There are numerous scientific studies that show a positive attitude helps a person overcome illness. There is almost unanimous agreement that the state of your mind has a great effect on the state of your body. More doctors are recognizing this fact and are starting to emphasize a more holistic approach toward treatment. Two of the books I read on the relationship between mind and body during this time were

There's a Lot More to Health than Not Being Sick by Bruce Larson and *Love, Medicine, and Miracles* by Bernie Siegel.

It has been said the best way to *be positive* is to *act positive*. It is difficult to act positive all the time. But the more you do it, the better off you will be.

There are a number of authors that can help you develop a positive attitude, even with your problems. Not all of these authors offer a complete view of Christian theology, but they certainly do a good job in the important element of promoting a positive attitude. These authors include Norman Vincent Peale, Og Mandino, and Robert Schuller.

The Crystal Cathedral in Garden Grove, California (Robert Schuller's church) has a statue of Job that I have stared at for hours throughout the years. I even have a paperweight with a chip of marble from that statue that was saved as the statue was being carved. I also have a keychain from the Crystal Cathedral with the *Possibility Thinker's Creed* by Robert Schuller:

> *When faced with a mountain, I will not quit. I will keep on striving until I climb over, find a pass through, tunnel underneath, or simply stay and turn the mountain into a gold mine, with God's help!*

Staying at Sloan-Kettering also taught me some lessons about what to expect from friends. When I was first in the hospital in Cincinnati, there were ten or fifteen people who flew from the east coast to visit me in Cincinnati. I was overwhelmed. I remember every time I heard the song *That's What Friends are For* (which was popular at the time), I got tears in my eyes. Four months later in New York, where I was a two hour drive from most of my friends, almost nobody came.

I might have surmised that I'm just not very popular, but I have talked to a lot of other people that have gone through a long sickness and the trend is almost exactly the same. In the beginning, everybody is visiting and sending cards. One month later, the only ones left are family, church people, and a few select friends.

I learned not to be disappointed by the lack of response from friends. Everyone is busy, and it's tough to show concern month after month. It taught me to value my family and church relationships even more. Judging from how people respond, family and church friends are the relationships that endure and should be cultivated. In fact, when I wrote this book, one of my best sources of the chronology (since I have a very bad memory) was the prayer update that my parents' church published every week. There were many other prayer chains going on for me at that time as well.

One other memory of my stay at Sloan-Kettering was meeting a volunteer who had been diagnosed with terminal cancer over ten years before. He had melanoma. When he was diagnosed, the doctors gave him four months to live (sound familiar?). When I met him, he was spending one day a week visiting cancer patients. I only talked to him for about five minutes, but just knowing that someone had overcome the same prognosis that I was given meant a lot to me.

My last memory of my hospital stay was playing a mean joke on my roommate. When you read this, you'll know why I had no friends. He checked in three days after me for chest surgery. He was Hispanic and spoke very little English, but we became friends and did our best to communicate.

Excerpts from the Faith Missionary Church
Wednesday night prayer requests

Jan. 22, 1986: GAVIN SINCLAIR - Son of Frank and Myrle is staying with his in-laws in Cincinnati, Ohio. Please continue to pray for successful treatment. Special prayer is being held for Gavin this evening at 6:30 p.m.

Feb. 5, 1986: There is no change at this point. The radiation, which he is tolerating very well, will be extended for two more weeks. Pray for his wife, Jennifer.

Feb. 19,1986: The radiation treatment ends this week. Doctors are hoping to take the tracheostomy tube out. This would be a big plus for Gavin. No change in the tumor at this point. Jennifer, his wife, is doing well. (Baby due in April.)

March 12, 1986: No update, but continue praying.

March 26, 1986: No change, but Gavin has doctor's appointment tomorrow regarding results of last x-ray.

Everyone on my floor was there for chest surgery. We all went through about the same process. We would be "prepped" for surgery the first day. The next day we would be in the operating room and then the recovery room. On the third day we would get back to our rooms, and the "evil" nurses would make us get up and walk around. Every night they would wake us up in the middle of the night to cough to clear out our chests. As I explained earlier, the surgeon would put in two chest tubes at the end of the surgery to collect any drainage that would collect in the days following the surgery. After four or five days, the drainage would be over and they would pull out the tubes. Another two or three days and you were ready to go home.

Pulling out the tubes was an interesting experience. When they pulled out the tubes, you could swear they had pulled out your lungs and heart as well. For a couple of moments, it was the most intense pain you can imagine.

My roommate was in surgery when I had my chest tubes pulled. The day I was going to leave, the residents came to pull the tubes on my friend. He was very nervous, and he motioned to me and said "Hurt?" What was I to do? Of course I told him "*no problema!*" He seemed satisfied and had this confident look on his face when they pulled the curtain between our rooms. A couple of seconds later he let out the most blood curdling scream I ever heard. When they pulled the curtain back, he looked at me and screamed, "You said no hurt!" I just laughed, and then he started laughing too (well, after *a while* he started laughing). As I said, you had better try to find humor in all the torture you go through!

Some people would say (quite reasonably) that this story sounds more cruel than funny. To an outsider, this is absolutely true. To a successful patient, this story is nothing. Successful patients can laugh at almost anything. I read about one lady on chemotherapy who thought it was hilarious when her wig fell into the chip dip at a party. Amputees routinely take out their fake limbs and swing them around for fun. Erma Bombeck wrote a good book on how children with cancer were able to find humor in their situation called *I Want to Grow Hair, I Want to Grow Up, I Want to Go to Boise* (see *Further Reading*). If you can't laugh at yourself and what you're going through, you are going to have problems.

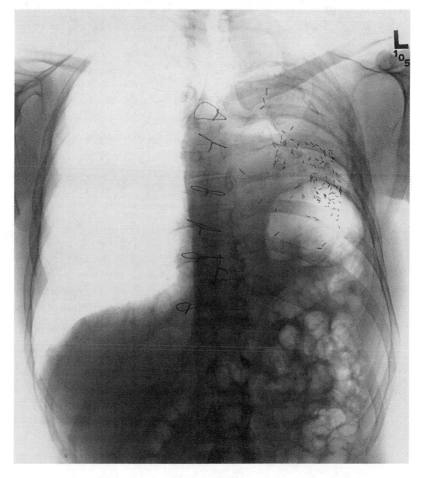

X-ray after surgery. Notice the wires wrapped around the chest bone and the radioactive seeds in the chest.

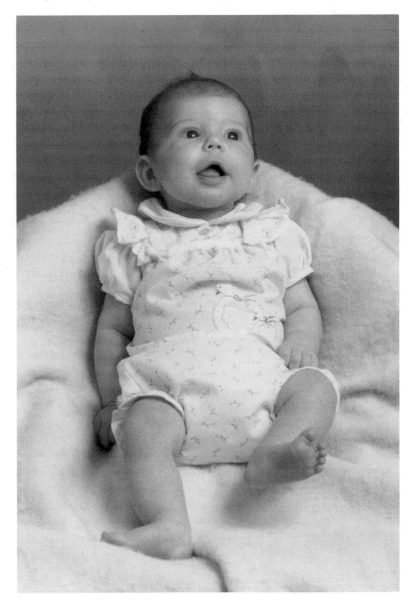

The new baby

Chapter 5: Parenthood

I was released from Memorial Sloan-Kettering one week before the baby was born. Jennifer and I made a good couple. She was incapacitated from being nine months pregnant, and I was incapacitated from having major chest surgery. I remember driving to the drug store one day, and neither one of us wanted to go in.

"You go in," Jennifer said. "I'm nine months pregnant."

"I can't go in," I countered. "I just had half of my insides ripped out." I think Jennifer ended up going in, because she is a lot tougher than I am.

Some men have sympathy pains when their wife becomes pregnant, actually getting morning sickness and cravings. I told everyone that I took things a bit too far by growing something inside my body just like my wife. "The ultimate in sympathy pains," I told everyone.

Finally, the big day came, and we went to the hospital. We had taken Lamaze classes, but based on my general incompetence in these things, Jennifer had gotten a back-up coach, our next-door-neighbor Charlotte. I had used the convenient excuse that I was too sick to be the coach.

I had to wear a lead vest because of the radioactive seeds in my chest. Unfortunately for Jennifer, most of the doctors that came in were more interested in the sickly-looking guy with the lead vest rather than the pregnant woman. Eventually Charlotte coached Jennifer through the delivery, and we had a baby girl who we named Jennette Nicole Sinclair. I was glad that I had lived to see her born, and now I could fill in the "Dear _____ " with "Dear Jennette." And maybe I could live long enough to tell her all the stories in person.

We brought the baby home from the hospital two days later. Jennifer's mother had come to New Jersey to help her. The days were both very happy and very sad. They were very happy, of course, because I had lived to see Jennette born. They were sad because I was totally unable to deal with her arrival.

One of the saddest times for me was when I was alone with Jennette once and she started to cry in her crib. I tried to pick her up but I couldn't physically do it. I was too weak from the surgery, and when I tried to pick her up it stretched my incision. She lay in the crib and cried, and I sat next to the crib on the floor and cried. I had so looked forward to the baby before she was born. Now that she had arrived, I found myself in a situation where I was totally useless.

After Jennifer's mother left, it was even harder on Jennifer. Because of my illness, she had missed out on the exciting time of being pregnant for the first time. Now she was home with a new baby and a husband who had just had major surgery, not to mention her responsibilities as a graduate student at Princeton. Somehow, we all survived.

Having my own child made me realize what it must be like to see your child suffer. The prognosis and treatment in Cincinnati had been very hard on my parents. During that time, I was much more worried about them than myself. I think it is harder to stand by and watch a loved one go through suffering than to go through it yourself. From a religious standpoint, through my father's suffering I began to understand why God sending His only Son to die on the cross was, in fact, the ultimate sacrifice. I asked my parents to write down what they were thinking during the first four months after I was diagnosed with terminal cancer. Some of the same details that I wrote about are repeated, but I think it is interesting to see the perspective of the parents compared to the patient.

From my mother:

It was December 27, 1985, when I received the call from Gavin. He was calling from Cincinnati where he was visiting his in-laws. He asked if I was sitting down. I thought he was just being funny and thought nothing of it. Then he said an x-ray he had taken for a bad cough had shown a tumor.

After hanging up the phone in the kitchen, I walked into the family room and told my sister Marjorie, my niece Maureen, and my husband Frank the news. Needless to say, I could hardly get it out and immediately burst into tears.

From my father:

Gavin called from Cincinnati and told Myrle the x-ray showed a tumor. I was standing in the doorway to the family room, and Myrle said it was all so sad. Marjorie and Maureen were wondering what to say or do at this dreadful time. I decided to go to Cincinnati the next morning. When I arrived, Jennifer and Jerry (Jennifer's father) gave me the details that I seemed not to hear.

Gavin walked into the downstairs family room, and I kissed the side of his face. We prayed that God would lead Gavin back to a normal life. Gavin and I left for his doctor appointment. Once again, I did not seem to hear the conversation.

After we came back from the doctor's appointment, I decided to call my daughter Mareth to tell her the news. When I started to talk, I broke down, so Gavin explained the tumor to his sister. I realized then how strong Gavin was during this terrible situation. At 3:30 p.m. on December 28, 1985, Gavin was admitted to Providence Hospital in Cincinnati.

We stayed in Cincinnati for several days. Mareth and her son, Corbin, came to join us. I remember one day Gavin came down from his room in a wheelchair to see Corbin. Gavin held his hand to his eyes and played peek with Corbin. This was typical of the attitude he would have for many years to come amidst all these circumstances. On New Year's Eve at 4 p.m., Dr. Morgan told us more details about Gavin's cancer. For me, a complete night's sleep was difficult.

From my mother:

Even without knowing the type of tumor, the doctors started Gavin on radiation on January 3, 1986. On January 6, not only did he have radiation but he also had a chemotherapy treatment. Just reading the literature on chemotherapy was chilling. They gave the treatment to him in the evening, and he was very sick the next day. Even so, he still received radiation every day except weekends.

On Saturday the 11th, they changed the diagnosis from thymoma to malignant fibrous hystiocytoma (sarcoma). This was literally a death sentence. After Dr. Morgan explained the situation, Gavin asked "How long?" The reply was four months. I left the room immediately and dissolved into tears. Kay, Dr. Morgan's nurse, put her arm around me. I remember Jennifer's mother coming from work because Jennifer had called her after getting the news. We just all sat around the waiting room not talking but each deep in our own private thoughts and prayers. Jennifer told us that Gavin wanted to be alone.

From my father:

The door to Gavin's hospital room was closed. Dr. Morgan had told me not to go in because Gavin was crying. I walked towards the elevator and Jennifer's mother gave me a hug. No conversation. My mind was whirling. I thought about Gavin a long time.

My memories went back to when Gavin was a small boy and all the things that we had experienced together:

* church league football, Gavin was "Big" number 77

* teaching Gavin a Windsor knot on a tie

* his one-eighth size violin

* his love for golf

This unstructured series of random thoughts filled my mind for many hours that afternoon and evening. Gavin's humor came through very strongly concerning his chemotherapy treatments. He told me (since I have a bald patch on the top of my head) that at least *his* hair would return. I also remember vividly Gavin's smile at the escorts taking him to have radiation. His humor seemed unstoppable.

Getting back to work was a rugged chore. My teary eyes would prevent seeing my typesetting work on my computer thinking about the future without Gavin. Without the concern of fellow workers, 8-5 would have been a nightmare. I would rerun memory films of "yesterdays" and Gavin became a total consuming force. Listening to music became too difficult because of constant reminders of past joys. Friends at our church, Faith Missionary, and the prayer group led by Pastor John Crocker on Wednesday evenings were the beginning of a breakthrough from the darkness of my spirit. The First Book of Samuel, Chapter 1, verse 11 has Hannah bargaining with God:

"If You do this, I will do this." I could not agree with this approach. One morning very early, after much sobbing, I knelt in front of our blue living room sofa and gave Gavin to God, life or death, and I told God that I would accept His will. Life continued to be difficult but bearable.

From my mother:

The period during Gavin's radiation treatments was especially difficult. Our prayer request was for the tumor to shrink, but the tumor was as big as ever.

A special prayer service was held at our church for Gavin on January 22. What marvelous support we had, not only from our church but also our friends and relatives. It was a very moving and joyous experience.

On February 22, Frank and I went over to Cincinnati with a rented van to load up their things for the trip back to Flemington, New Jersey. Among the articles were new things for the expectant baby. The next day we left in the van and Gavin and Jennifer left in their car. It was bittersweet. We had been so close to them geographically while they were in Cincinnati, and that would end. On the other hand, Gavin was eager to return home, not to mention Jennifer, who needed to get back to her graduate work at Princeton University. Can you imagine having a husband in the hospital with inoperable cancer and you in graduate school and pregnant?

Frank and I went with Gavin and Jennifer to his appointment at Sloan-Kettering on March 22 for an exam, consultation, and x-ray. He had to return the next day for a heart test. The drive from Flemington to New York City via the Holland Tunnel was already getting very familiar.

Frank and I went back to Indianapolis on April 1. Gavin's x-ray on April 6 showed a little shrinkage of the tumor. On April 8 Gavin had an appointment with a surgeon. Gavin called to say that he was scheduled for surgery on Mon-

day and Dr. Barnes would try to remove the tumor. Frank left immediately (6:30 p.m.) for New Jersey. He took Gavin to Sloan-Kettering on April 10 for admission. I flew in to Newark, New Jersey the next day and both Frank and I went to see Gavin. We visited, along with Jennifer, the next two days and Gavin was very upbeat about the coming surgery. What did he have to lose?

Monday morning, April 14, the three of us left for the hospital at 4 a.m. When we arrived they told us we couldn't see Gavin then, but at 6:30 we saw him until they took him to surgery at 7 a.m. The surgery lasted from 8 a.m. to 2 p.m. Someone from the hospital would update all the families hourly and answer any questions. I am sure that everyone started looking for the "update lady" before the hour was up. I was very calm and very optimistic. I knew hundreds of people were praying, most of whom had never met Gavin. It was in God's hands.

I think it was between 3 and 4 that Dr. Barnes came to the waiting room to tell us that the surgery had gone well. The tumor had been removed and also one lung and the sac around the heart. Dr. Barnes implanted 106 radioactive seeds next to the ribs. We had many questions that Jennifer had written down. He very kindly sat down and answered all of them for us. We sailed out of the hospital, after making numerous phone calls, to a "beautiful" New York City. Some memories have faded but not that one. Our drive to Flemington was on the "wings of eagles."

My parents clearly had a difficult time during this period. When Jennette was born, I could relate even more. It is much easier to go through an illness yourself than to watch your child suffer. I am now a total wreck whenever I watch a movie about parents and a sick child. I think *Lorenzo's Oil* is the saddest movie I've ever watched. I am sorry I put my parents through all this, but I think they got through the experience with a deeper understanding of life. My dad had prostate cancer in 1993, and he says my experience helped him prepare for his own battle with cancer. I'll now continue the story that left off after Jennette was born.

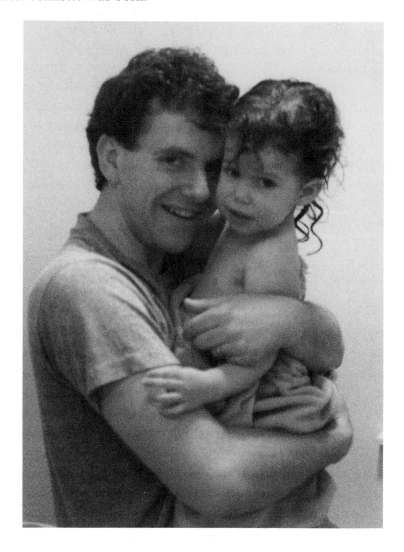

Jennette and her dad

Chapter 6: The Darkest Days

About a month after Jennette was born, I returned to Sloan-Kettering for a Teflon injection to my vocal cord. This surgery brought my two vocal cords closer together and improved the quality of my voice. Even better, the doctors at Sloan-Kettering said I didn't need any more chemotherapy. For the first time in months, things really started looking better. My voice had returned to a functional level. I began making plans for my return to work. I started to feel in control again.

While I was planning how many weeks it would be before I could return to work, I got a sharp reminder to be more humble and recognize how fragile and precarious human life really is.

Three days after the Teflon injection, I woke up one night with a fever of 104 degrees. I was immediately admitted to the local hospital where I was treated for pneumonia. I did not respond to treatment. In fact, my fever increased to 106 degrees at one point. The fever caused seizures, and a couple of times I lost all muscular control over my body.

My experience at this hospital was one of the worst weeks of my life. It seemed that the staff at the hospital had no idea what they were doing. My main doctor seemed to diagnose "Legionnaire's Disease" for every patient. Even though I was getting more experienced with doctors and the hospital scene, I was still reluctant to tell the doctors at the local hospital that I was leaving to seek help elsewhere. One thing I eventually overcame was not feeling badly when I told a doctor I wanted to get a second opinion, or that I would rather get my treatment elsewhere. But it was my body and my money (or at least my insurance company's money), and I had to do what I thought was best.

Even more frightening was knowing this would have been the hospital I would have gone to for my cancer treatments had my family doctor in New Jersey correctly diagnosed my problem in the beginning. I probably would have stayed there, not knowing enough to investigate other options. The experience at this hospital made me even more sure that *all things work for good*, and it was a real blessing that I was not diagnosed with cancer until I got to Cincinnati.

The doctors at the local hospital could not diagnose my illness, and I finally found the courage to say I was leaving. The final straw came when they decided they would try to put a tube through my nose and down into the lung to try to suction out the fluid they thought was in my lung. An orderly came in with a tube and a pump. He was wearing a "Grateful Dead" T-shirt (not a good sign) and an unbuttoned white coat. He tried to shove the tube into my nose and down through the airway to the lung, but all he ended up doing was perforating my septum (i.e., he put a hole through the inside of my nose between the two nostrils).

I packed up and headed back to see my surgeon at Sloan-Kettering. After a week of observation at Sloan-Kettering, they could not identify the problem. They sent me home with the hope that the problem would clear up by itself. Here's how I described the situation in a letter to a relative in Canada:

> *I was doing fine through the surgery and the Teflon injection to my vocal cords, then the problems began. Several days after my "non-stick throat" procedure, I started running fevers up to 106 degrees. I checked into my local hospital, where my doctor decided I had Legionnaire's disease. Why he thought that, I'm not so sure. He started me on intravenous antibiotics that systematically destroyed one vein per day. It felt like I was mainlining sulfuric acid.*
>
> *Next, another doctor entered the scene who wanted to do CT scans of my brain. I know a bad trend when I see one, so I went back to Sloan-Kettering. At Sloan-Kettering they took blood and checked my temperature every day, but they never figured out what was wrong with me. After a week of that, I went home.*

Whenever I wasn't sure what to do, I went back to the doctor I had the most confidence in, Dr. Morgan in Cincinnati. You always need one doctor who can be the quarterback. My situation was a little more complicated because I had received treatment in three different cities by that time, but I always did my best to send all the records to Dr. Morgan so he could see the big picture.

When I told Dr. Morgan about my situation over the phone, he feared that a tumor might be present that was causing the problem. I decided to return to Cincinnati for more chemotherapy. Before they could give me the chemotherapy treatment, however, the doctor who administered my radiation in Cincinnati checked me over. He thought the fevers might be caused by inflammation from the radiation several months earlier. He was right. Steroids eliminated the problem in only a couple of days.

This brings up another point about doctors. Over twenty doctors had evaluated my condition looking for the cause of the high fevers. I had blood tests, a bronchoscopy (where they looked inside my bronchial tubes and lungs for blockages or tumors), and lots of poking and probing. Generally, doctors look for a cause that fits their specialty. They evaluate the symptoms, and then match the symptoms to the diseases they know about. This is a good reason for seeking many opinions on your problem. Different specialists recommend different treatments based on their particular experience.

When Dr. Morgan and I were discussing what had happened to me since I left Cincinnati, he said he was very surprised that Sloan-Kettering had done the operation on me. "Well, I guess you don't get a hit unless you go to bat," he quipped.

Even though the steroids fixed the fever and there were no more signs of cancer, Dr. Morgan thought some precautionary chemotherapy treatments would be wise. Jennifer and Jennette went back to New Jersey after the chemotherapy treatment since Jennifer had already missed a lot of school, and I stayed in Cincinnati with my in-laws.

Those days in Cincinnati were some of the longest days of my life. I was wiped out from the chemotherapy (as usual), and my wife and daughter were back in New Jersey. The only thing in my favor was the textured ceiling in my room–you can see a lot of animals in the swirls if you stare long enough.

It's interesting what enters an empty mind. I knew a few Bible verses, and they would sometimes pop into my brain. More often I would hear jingles from commercials. This was another one of those things that made it clear I had been living my life with the wrong priorities.

I fell into bad habits, lying around during the day, sleeping on and off. During the night, I couldn't sleep because I had lain around all day. I should have forced myself to be more active and maintain a normal cycle. I was now on my eighth month of treatment, and I thought I would have been back at work by this time. I was depressed because of feeling so terrible and being away from my family.

About three weeks after my chemotherapy treatment, I went back to see Dr. Morgan for a check-up and to discuss future treatment. I had already decided I didn't want any more chemotherapy, which was a source of disagreement between me and everyone else who cared about me. From an outside perspective, more chemotherapy made sense. I was getting through it, and chemotherapy could certainly help kill any cancer cells.

I had a very inside perspective, mostly the inside of my guts (literally). I had decided no more chemotherapy. Period.

This is another fine line issue. I am not sure treatment does any good if the patient is totally against it. On the other hand, it makes sense to get the best medical treatment possible and take advantage of all the different treatments. This is one to work out on a case-to-case basis, but I don't think anyone should go into the decision thinking that one view is automatically right. In my case, there was no evidence of any cancer. If the x-rays had still shown a tumor, I probably would have gladly gone ahead with more chemotherapy. In the book *Cancer...there's hope*, Richard and Annette Bloch make the strong argument that it is better to be safe than sorry.

Fortunately, Dr. Morgan saved the day and said he didn't think more chemotherapy was necessary. My cancer treatments were finally over, and I returned home to New Jersey.

I had lost twenty pounds from the last chemotherapy treatment. I gradually gained back the weight, and I will tell you how if you promise not to report me to any nutritionist group.

Almost everyone with cancer has problems keeping up their weight. I'm told that malnutrition is actually the cause of death for many seriously ill people. It is a real problem that must be addressed. I don't necessarily recommend my method of gaining weight for everyone, so take this with a large grain of salt.

The first thing I did was forget about this "well-balanced diet" stuff. If you are having problems gaining weight, getting calories is the principal objective. Cancer is very disruptive to your eating patterns. Many foods will seem repulsive. I absolutely could not eat red meat during my cancer treatment and for two years thereafter. I alternated between hating milk and loving milk for three years. I finally came to the conclusion that I was going to go through "fads" in my eating habits. I ate certain things almost exclusively until that food didn't appeal to me anymore, and then I moved on to something else. I'm sure nutritionists are cringing at this, but a well-balanced meal that is not eaten doesn't do much good.

One of my binges was Nestles Crunch Bars and milk. I ate those for three months. Another was Long John Silver's fish meals. One good thing about these binges is they were high in calories. A head lettuce binge is not going to help much. I accepted the fact that my taste buds were totally con-fused, and I concentrated more on eating something with calo-ries rather than worrying too much about whether it was "good for me" or not. For a different, and infinitely more sensible, approach to nutrition, you may want to read *A Cancer Battle Plan*, by Anne and David Frähm.

There are a number of nutritional supplements available on the market. During my many hospital stays, I noticed that these options were getting better and better. Sometimes people could fool me by sneaking high energy powders into my food. If these powders were added in low quantities, I didn't notice them. The problem is that people try to load too much in, and that can be a permanent turn-off.

Scheduling an exercise period before and after eating can be helpful. Part of my normal routine in the hospital was to do laps around the hospital corridors before and after each meal. Lying in bed before and after eating does nothing for your appetite or digestion.

I remember the time between the Teflon injection at Sloan-Kettering and leaving Cincinnati after recovering from the last bout of chemotherapy as the worst time in the entire treatment. In the first few months of my cancer treatments, at least there was a lot happening. There were decisions to make on various treatments, and there were new medical tests that I had never experienced. It was almost interesting, in a perverse sort of way. During the period after the Teflon injection, it seems that all I did was lie around and suffer. I didn't remember exactly how bad this period was until I read how my mother described it.

From my mother:

Had only four months elapsed since the cancer surgery at Sloan-Kettering? It felt like four years. I received many painful phone calls from Gavin during that time, especially late at night. He was feeling so terrible. I would get off the phone and cry, not only because I was unable to do anything, but also because he was in so much pain. His after-surgery problems were daunting. My jubilation was turning to gloom. Only by reminding myself that he was alive was I able to go on with my life, such as it was at that time.

Frank, Gavin's grandma, and I arrived in Flemington on May 23 to see Jennette for the first time. What a joy. What a good baby. Unfortunately, this was offset by Gavin, who was feeling badly and in no way contributed to our joy. He had a lead vest that he wore when he was going to be close to anyone, especially Jennette, but his vain efforts to hold the baby were pitiful. He basically wanted to be left alone in his misery, and at that point I thought I could never be sadder. We concentrated on our new granddaughter.

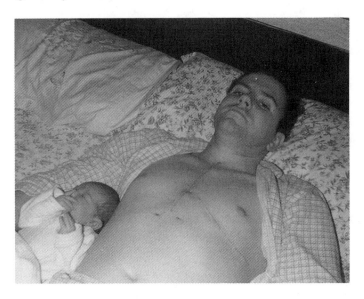

Gavin and Jennette

Gavin made an unexpected trip to the local hospital on June 2. The doctors were at a loss to diagnose the problem. They thought pneumonia, Legionnaire's disease, cancer? All Gavin wanted to do was get out of there and go to Memorial Sloan-Kettering, which he did on June 9. The following day they did a bronchoscopy and it looked like pneumonia. Then they said it was not pneumonia but possibly an infectious disease. The final diagnosis was a staph and yeast infection. Later we would discover that this was not correct either.

I visited Gavin at Sloan-Kettering on June 14. Gavin looked worse than I had ever seen him before. In a mere whisper he said "I have to get out of here. They are killing me." He not only looked terrible but he was not himself mentally. They were sending him home the next day.

I stayed for a week and the memories still haunt me. It appeared that Gavin had given up. He wasn't eating, he wasn't communicating, he stayed in bed, and he popped pain pills like candy. I don't think I will ever forget him sitting on the porch, looking so forlorn, as Jennifer drove me to the bus that would take me to Newark airport for my trip home. It seemed like we stopped in twenty towns en route and I cried through every one, as well as in between.

Gavin, Jennifer, and Jennette all flew to Cincinnati for an appointment with Dr. Morgan. Gavin had a bone scan and x-ray at the hospital and visited the nurses who had cared for him earlier that year. I'm sure the Cincinnati people had not expected to see him alive, unless the grapevine was working.

On July 30 I went over to Cincinnati to look after Jennette while Jennifer took Gavin to his chemotherapy treatment. Jennifer had to get her mother to help her get Gavin back into the house when they got back. He could not walk on his own and struggled up the stairs to the bedroom. Gavin made some remark to me, but I was so distraught at seeing him looking so badly, I had no idea what he said.

Jennifer and Jennette went back to Flemington the next day. I returned the next day to be with Gavin since his in-laws would be working. Thus began a couple more trips to Cincinnati for Frank and me.

Gavin went home to Flemington on August 16 with the good news of no more chemotherapy.

We should not feel like we have failed if we can't remain positive all the time. I felt guilty for my feelings during this time until I remembered that even Jesus, during his darkest hour on the cross, called out, "My God, My God. Why have You forsaken me?"

While we may not be able to be positive all the time, we should try to make these periods short and recognize that it's during these really tough times when we need God the most.

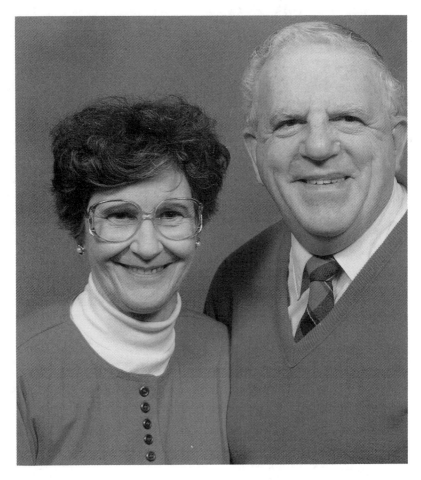

Frank and Myrle Sinclair

Chapter 7: Back to Work

After two months of further recuperation, I was ready to return to work. I arranged a schedule where I would work four days a week, taking one day per week for doctor appointments, physical and voice therapy.

The first time back into my office was strange. First of all, many of my books were gone. I guess when people heard I was going to die, they didn't wait for the reading of the will to see if they were going to inherit my books! Instead, people had just taken them. (I worked with very aggressive people.)

The other thing about getting back to work was being with normal people again. After months of being in hospitals and doctors' offices, you lose perspective. If you have a coughing fit in a hospital, nobody pays any attention. Try it in a business meeting, however, and people think you have malaria.

People had a hard time knowing how to treat me. Many were afraid of saying the wrong thing. What they didn't know was I had already heard it all. They didn't need to worry about offending me. One of my favorite stories came during one of those "discussions around the coffee machine." A group of guys was planning to play basketball that evening. One of them asked me, "Gavin, do you want to come and play basketball?" One of my friends whispered to him, loudly enough that everyone could hear, "That's not nice. You know Gavin only has one lung." Without missing a beat, the other guy said, "Well, we could play half court."

Getting back in the mainstream forced me to get better. It took my mind off my feelings of nausea and pain and made me push forward. A few months before, when I was lying in bed day after day with the pain from my operation, Jennifer came in (frustrated at dealing with a one-month-old baby) and told me I was useless. I thought she was the meanest person in the world. "To call me useless after all I had been through," I thought. It wasn't until five years later that I realized this was exactly what I needed to hear.

There is a fine line between caring for a person and babying them too much. If you are the patient, you need to recognize at some point you need to get up and do something, even if you don't feel like it. And once you start, you realize that you can do it. Getting back in the mainstream distracts you from your pain and problems, forces you to become more active, which in turn makes you feel better. I just feel sorry for the person (my wife in this case) who has to tell the patient to quit whining and get back into the game.

My biggest ongoing problem after returning to work was pain. I did all the physical therapy with no results. I tried a TENS unit, which is a little box that sends electrical impulses into your body. The idea is that the external electrical impulses confuse the pain impulses traveling through the nervous system. That didn't work, but it sure did feel weird, kind of like sticking your finger into an electrical outlet. I also tried every drug imaginable. Narcotic drugs were the only thing that gave me any relief.

With the aid of the narcotic drugs, I could carry on a fairly normal life. I played with my daughter. In fact, I spoiled her rotten. I did my job, traveling a lot to Europe and especially South America. Before my cancer diagnosis, I had focused my professional life on positioning myself for the next promotion at work. After my illness, I learned to appreciate every day for itself. I did my best and tried to enjoy what I was doing every day. With my new attitude, I ended up getting three promotions in two years.

Jennifer finished at Princeton, and we moved from Flemington, New Jersey to Bethlehem, Pennsylvania in June 1988. This was closer to my job in Allentown, Pennsylvania and Jennifer's new job at Lafayette College in Easton, Pennsylvania. I resumed work at night on my master's degree in economics at Lehigh University.

Another thing Jennifer and I started thinking about was having another child. The first one had turned out so well, we thought another one would be good. Unfortunately, the chemotherapy had done nothing for my manliness. My sperm count was only about 10 million, compared to a normal of 70 million. Other than the fertility problem and my continuing pain, everything was pretty good.

The only times that were a little tense was when I had to go in for cancer check-ups. I had to have an x-ray every three months at first. Then it was stretched out to every six months and finally once a year. Since my cancer was an aggressive type, my doctors said if it didn't come back quickly it was probably gone. Every x-ray was clean. Each check-up got easier and easier. I thought my problems were over.

Chapter 8: Congestive Heart Failure

After two years of clear check-ups I had almost forgotten about cancer. I was beginning to think I was normal. My body started to rebel in August 1988. I started getting that nauseous feeling again, just like when I was diagnosed with cancer the first time.

Recurrence is a scary feeling for someone who has had cancer. I went back to Cincinnati to see the doctors that I trusted the most. It was almost like reliving the experience again. First I went to see Dr. Richards, and he examined me with a worried look on his face. He spent a long time feeling my liver to see if it was enlarged. I remember crying, not from pain but thinking that he had found cancer again.

I was sent back to the hospital for tests, just like the first time. My 95-year-old grandmother in Indianapolis died when I was in the hospital. This was another very difficult time for my father. His mother had just died and I was back in the hospital, possibly with cancer again.

The first thing they did to me in the hospital was a MUGA scan, which was an unknown test to me. (MUGA is an

71

abbreviation for "multi-gated acquisition," whatever that means.) To do this test, the technicians gave me a radioactive injection, and then they scanned my heart. The test told how efficiently my heart was pumping out blood, measured as an "ejection fraction." Why they were checking my heart, I wasn't really sure. Before I went to the next test, a CT scan, Dr. Morgan met me in the hallway of the hospital. "Never mind with the CT scan," he told me. "We found the problem."

According to the MUGA scan, my heart was only working at 50% of normal. That resulted in a fluid build-up, which in turn caused nausea and swelling. Dr. Morgan, the chemotherapy doctor, said the heart problems were probably caused by the radiation. The next day I saw my radiation doctor, and he said the heart problems were probably caused by the chemotherapy. I tried to avoid getting these two guys in the same room, because I didn't want a fight. It didn't matter to me whether the heart problem was caused by the chemotherapy or the radiation. Both treatments had a part in destroying the cancer and saving my life.

Even though I had serious problems with my heart, I was very encouraged when the problem was identified. It was always easier for me once I knew what the problem was, even if the problem was serious. I always thought the *known* was much easier to deal with than the *unknown*. Once you know what you are facing, it motivates the fighting instinct.

To confirm the results of the MUGA scan, I had a cardiac catheterization. This was a fascinating test. The doctors feed a line though an artery in the leg, and then they move the line through the veins until they get to the heart. Using this procedure, they can measure various pressures at different points in the heart. You can watch the whole test on a television monitor. Unfortunately, I couldn't see very well without my glasses. I didn't like the initial insertion of the tube into the artery and when they fed the tube into the vein, because it gave me a weird rubbing feeling. Otherwise, it was an interesting test.

The cardiac catheterization confirmed the results from the MUGA scan. The doctors put me into the hospital and gave me diuretics to decrease the fluid level in my body. When the heart is not working efficiently, the body builds up fluids. Diuretics take off the excess fluid.

It's sometimes hard to see the effect of certain drugs. One hour after taking Lasix, the diuretic, I was "expelling" pints of fluid. It was undoubtedly the most effective drug I had ever taken, at least in terms of "measurable" effect. The doctors also put me on Digoxin, a drug to make the heart beat stronger, and Capoten, a drug to decrease the back pressure on the heart. I was released from the hospital feeling very well.

The next trick I had to learn was when to take my daily Lasix. Like clockwork, one hour after taking the pill I had to be close to a bathroom. Miscalculations were either embarrassing or painful. If I took the pill too close to a meeting, I had to ex-cuse myself every ten minutes throughout the meeting. That tends to draw attention to oneself. That was the embarrassing part. Once I took the pill before leaving a hotel for the Los Angeles airport, and I found myself stuck in a traffic jam. That was the painful part.

Another difficult experience was an MRI scan (magnetic resonance imaging) that was done on my heart. The MRI was not a new test for me. I had several over the previous years. An MRI takes a very clear image, much better than an x-ray or CT scan. It operates with magnets, and there is no radiation involved. The bad part of a MRI is they put you in a tube slightly bigger than your body and close you up, not unlike packing a sardine in a can. The technician gives you instructions through a speaker inside the tube. An MRI would be a good screening tool for finding able-bodied people for submarine duty, because if you are the slightest bit claustrophobic, you find out quickly.

Usually an MRI only takes 15 minutes, and even that is too long for many people. I talked to several people that had to discontinue the test because it was unbearable for them. To diagnose my heart problem, the doctors wanted to put together a series of MRIs so they could reconstruct an entire cycle of my heart beat. I was in the tube for over two hours. I thought about what it would be like to be a POW again, thinking how glad I was there were no rats or snakes inside the tube.

Overall, the new combination of heart drugs kept me ticking pretty well. I still had pain, however, even though I had been taking morphine continuously for the past two years. That would lead to the next problem.

Chapter 9: Spinal Surgery

With the cancer apparently gone and my heart back in working order, you would have thought my problems were over. They were not. The thing I was left with was chronic pain. I don't know where the pain came from. It was in the left side of my chest, so it could have been the surgery or more likely the radiation. All I knew was it hurt all the time.

Ever since my cancer surgery I had dealt with the pain problem using narcotic drugs. I had tried many other options, including non-narcotic drugs, physical therapy, and the TENS unit. Nothing worked except the narcotic drugs. So I kept taking them, in higher and higher doses, until I became almost immune to the effect. I was experiencing less and less pain relief, even though I had built up to what would have been a lethal dose of morphine for a normal person. I felt like I was in a downward spiral. I was dependent on the drugs for survival, and I knew they would become increasingly less helpful.

When I looked back in my journal during this period I found many sad entries, most of them late at night when the pain was keeping me up. Here is an example:

January 20, 1989 (21st actually)
Friday night/Saturday morning
1:40 a.m.

> *Well, the pain is keeping me up tonight. Sometimes I feel like I'm at my breaking point. Jennifer and Jennette were late getting home tonight, and I started wondering (somewhat sadistically, I suppose) "what if" they had been killed in a car crash. Would I still want to be alive? Quite honestly, probably not. I have a very bad attitude when it comes to my pain. On every other subject, I can approach my trials and tribulations with a positive attitude. The pain is so bad it's taking over now. I am driven because Jennette and Jennifer need me.*

One of the problems with pain is that it takes away your initiative to fight. It is difficult to focus on anything—mentally, physically, or spiritually—if you are in great pain. Chronic pain is especially difficult. Most phases of treatment have a time period. An operation comes to an end. A test comes to an end. Chronic pain may never end, and that is a much more difficult challenge.

Another problem with pain is it lies on the boundary between the physical and the mental. If you have a tumor, it can easily be shown on an x-ray. There is no question that you have a tumor. With pain, it is not always easy to show that it physically exists. Some people start thinking they should be able to "tough it out," that maybe it is all mental, or some other feeling based on the fact that physical evidence is not available. Even worse, in some cases friends or family may think you are not really in that much pain, and they may be less sensitive to your pain problem than they are with your more definitive problems.

Finally, pain can have a snowballing effect. Once you start to experience pain, you may compensate by adjusting your posture or reducing your physical activity, both of which can increase the pain even more.

With all of these problems in mind, the critical fact to remember is the pain problem *must be defeated*. There can be no recovery unless the pain problem is confronted and conquered. I got to the point where drastic measures were needed. Narcotics were simply not the answer if I was going to be living for a while. After seeing many different doctors, the best option seemed to be a nerve block.

A nerve block is an operation where the sensory nerves off the spinal cord are cut. The nerve block leaves you with no sensation in the area controlled by the severed nerves, just a totally numb feeling. But you can't feel pain in that area either. This is not a choice for everybody, because for some parts of the body the sensory and motor nerves are combined. If you cut one of these nerves, you lose both sensory and motor ability.

There are many nerves that run off the spinal cord, and the doctors selectively choose the ones to sever to numb the correct part of the body. These nerves are numbered, and the nerves in the thoracic area are T1-T12. In my case, severing the T2-T9 nerves would numb my left chest.

My doctors did a temporary block by injecting chemicals into the correct nerves. They essentially anesthetized the T2-T9 nerves to test if numbing the areas controlled by these nerves would give me relief from my pain. It was a very strange sensation, but the procedure helped the pain. I decided to go ahead with the surgery.

Once again, I returned to Cincinnati, the place where I felt the most comfortable. My mother can fill you in on what happened.

From my mother:

I dropped off Gavin and Frank and went to park the car. We all met at admitting. A volunteer came with a wheel chair and we all went to the twelfth floor. The doctors and nurses were flabbergasted at the thirty morphine pills per day that Gavin was taking. Six people came in to check and recheck the amount written in the history. After Gavin put on the hospital gown, he asked the nurse, "Do I look like a patient now?" The anesthesiologist came in and discussed the plans for surgery. Gavin had an x-ray and an EKG.

Gavin said to be at the hospital at 10 a.m. the next day as he would leave for surgery at about 11 a.m. Actually he left around 10:45 a.m., so we were excited that everything was going to be ahead of schedule. Frank and I went to the twelfth floor waiting room. After waiting awhile Frank went down to the sixth floor and found out that they had just put Gavin to sleep at approximately 2 p.m. So much for ahead of schedule. Time dragged on. Frank slept. We went to the sixth floor at 4 p.m. to check on progress. We waited on the sixth floor for the doctor. Uncle Eddie (Jennifer's uncle) came and we talked for about an hour. Uncle Eddie left and the surgeon came out at 6:40 p.m. He said, "It was quite an operation, but Gavin came through it very well." There was a backup of blood they hadn't anticipated. The doctor said they almost didn't continue. However, they knew Gavin would be very upset when he woke up in pain and they hadn't done anything. The surgeon told us they cut T2 to T10 (note: they had not intended to cut T10). The doctor told us Gavin would be up in the intensive care unit (ICU) at 8:30 p.m.

We went in to see Gavin at 8:30 p.m. and he had good color. But he was flat on his back and in an intense amount of pain. The nurse asked us for our phone number and gave us a direct number to call through the night. The surgeon and his assistants came in with a probe to check Gavin's left side. His left side was numb (which was expected) but also the inside of his left arm and two fingers on the left hand (which was not expected). Gavin didn't want us to stay. We talked to the doctors outside ICU. They said swelling could be causing the numbness in the arm and fingers, and the feeling could come back. We were very happy that it appeared there was no pain in the chest, although the pain in his back from the surgery was excruciating.

At the first visiting hour period of the next day, Gavin was in a lot of pain so we only stayed a short time. We came back at the next visiting time, and I fed Gavin three pieces of apple in his Waldorf salad. He looked pitiful. He was still in a lot of pain, but he could regulate the medication somewhat with a button connected to the IV. He had on leg massagers to prevent blood clots. He was sitting in a chair, but barely.

Frank and I left for Indianapolis about 8 p.m. I hated to leave. It reminded me of when I left Gavin in Flemington after being there for a week.

Handwritten note from my mother at bottom of her typed writing: *Gavin, you told me you were very frightened when you woke up in ICU. You hadn't expected that.*

Waking up after the spinal surgery was totally different than waking up from the cancer surgery. After the cancer surgery, I remember gradually waking up and gradually remembering why I was there. I was in very little pain. When waking up after the spinal surgery, all I remember was intense pain in my back. It literally felt like the doctors were still cutting directly into my back. Maybe it was because I had been taking so many pain pills, and after the surgery I remember they were scared to give me even as much as I had been taking normally before the surgery. If someone would have offered to put me out of my misery during that period in ICU, I would have gladly agreed. I remember having a battle of wills with the nurse. She told me to lie flat, but I kept moving my pillow behind me because my back hurt so badly. Finally the doctor came and said it would be all right if I sat up some. This was the only time I remember purposely doing something in direct disobedience to a nurse when I knew she was right. I felt badly later for giving her a hard time.

It turns out the numbness in my left hand was the result of cutting the T10 nerve, which was unintended. I spent about a week in the hospital recovering from the surgery. I was in more pain than ever, but I hoped the pain would go away when the incision healed. The doctors were not in agreement on what to do about the narcotic drugs. Some felt I should stay on them to help me recover from the surgery; others thought I should stop them in the hospital. The withdrawal symptoms from the narcotics would be intense, and stopping while in the hospital would be safer.

In this case, the doctors asked me what I wanted to do without giving a conclusion of their own. I opted for staying on the narcotics until I recovered from the surgery, and then weaning off them later. In retrospect, I don't know if that was the right decision.

I went home and started reducing my pill intake. As my incision healed, I started to feel better. I went from 30 pills a day to five pills a day fairly quickly. I was doing so well, I decided to go back to work. The left side of my chest felt pretty good. The only weird thing was taking a shower and not feeling the water against half of my body.

Going from five pills to zero was a bigger problem than I had thought. Whenever I cut down below five, I would get very bad withdrawal symptoms: nausea, fever, and cramps. Since I was now back at work, I could not do my job if I was having withdrawal symptoms. So I ended up staying at five pills a day, not because of pain but to control the withdrawal symptoms.

I was now in big trouble. The whole time I was taking the drugs for pain, I wondered if the problem was in my head. Now I knew the pain was gone, but I was still taking the pills. This disgusted me even more.

The story turns to where it gets so frustrating, it becomes funny again. To try to control the withdrawal symptoms, the doctor gave me Compazine, which is an anti-nausea drug. When I started taking the drug, not only did I feel as bad as ever, but I literally could not sit down. I had to keep walking around like a nervous little kid. The chemical factory in my body was really going crazy. When I saw the doctor, he explained this was a possible side effect of Compazine. In fact, the Nazis used to give Compazine to people in concentration camps to try to drive them crazy. It was certainly working on me. Needless to say, I stopped taking the Compazine.

During this time I was in the process of changing jobs and moving to a company in Pittsburgh. When I took the physical for my new job, I told them my medical history, including the fact that I was taking narcotic drugs. "No problem," the personnel person told me. "As long as you disclose the prescription drugs that you are taking, there is no problem on the drug test." Famous last words.

When the results came back positive on the drug test, the same personnel person told me they couldn't hire me until I was clean on the drug test. Meanwhile, I had told my previous employer that I was leaving, and Jennifer had a new job in Pittsburgh. We're talking high stress level now, especially on top of the original problem of withdrawal symptoms from the narcotic drugs.

When you are in trouble, you go back to the fundamentals. I had lost sight of the basics during all these problems. The pain had clouded my ability to concentrate on the right things. I went back to God for the answer. Through Him, I found the strength to overcome the withdrawal symptoms, pass the drug test, and move on with life.

When I was having the cancer treatments, I always came back to *all things work for good*. I didn't lose sight of the objective, because I automatically came back to that thought when facing any problem. I didn't come back to anything at first during my experience with pain, and I didn't do very well.

Many people have come to me with their problems with pain. The first thing I tell them is to fully explore all of the medical treatments available. Since no one completely understands the mechanism of pain, there are a wide variety of treatments available. One method may be great for one person, and totally worthless for another. You should keep trying until you find something that helps. Do not get discouraged if method after method is not successful. Since the method that may help you could be very specific, the fact that many methods may fail does not mean there is not something that will work for you. I went through fifteen or twenty different methods, ranging from strange concoctions of drugs to medical devices to physical therapy. Most of these methods had no effect. But I kept trying until I found something that would help me deal with my pain. If you have chronic pain, you need to do the same. There are many pain clinics that can introduce you to a wide variety of methods.

Although I am not qualified to review the wide variety of pain methods available, I would like to address one particular treatment area where I have a great deal of experience– narcotic drugs. Narcotic drugs are both the greatest thing and worst thing in the area of pain management. Narcotic drugs are very effective in controlling pain. Narcotic drugs can also plunge you into a never-ending trap of physical, and sometimes mental, dependency. This is compounded by the mental trauma of consuming substances that are regarded as evil substances in our society. Nowhere is the complicated interface between the physical and mental state more difficult than on the subject of narcotic drugs.

I found most doctors were not very helpful in dealing with the subject of narcotic drugs. I quickly learned that most doctors could be classified as narcotic Puritans, who believed that all narcotic drugs should be avoided, or narcotic Hedonists, who believed that any quantity of narcotics was acceptable.

The combination of a patient who is already worried about becoming a drug addict because he or she took Percocet after surgery and a narcotic Puritan for a doctor can be a devastating combination. One of my friends was in this situation. Guilt compounded the problem of pain, just making the situation worse.

To me, the clearest answer is to set a time limit on the use of narcotic drugs. In the short run, narcotic drugs are often the best solution to pain and give the body and mind a chance to recover. Just as clear to me is that narcotic drugs are not a long-term solution. Eventually the body becomes physically dependent on these drugs, and the withdrawal symptoms become yet another battle to fight.

The balance on this issue is critical. If you are dealing with chronic pain, you must first start with a clear conscience and decide that narcotic drugs will help you recover. At some point later, you must decide with equal conviction to switch to a long-term pain management program. The new program will probably not be nearly as effective as the way you were able to control your pain with narcotic drugs. After all, I had to have my nerves surgically disconnected from my spinal cord, which left me with numbness in my left side and sporadic, but not continuous, pain. But the fact is that narcotic drugs are not a long-term option.

Chapter 10: STROKE! (and a scare)

After I passed the drug test, we finally moved to Pittsburgh. I was in better shape than I had been in for years. The chronic pain was gone. I still had sharp, stabbing pains at times during the day, but that was tolerable.

As I looked for new doctors, I was glad I had assembled my own copies of key medical reports. I never trusted the filing systems of most hospitals and doctors. I think Sloan-Kettering is still looking for my stress test results. My personal copies of discharge reports, surgery reports, and other key medical records told my new doctors most of what they needed to know.

My new internist was very good and gave me some simple solutions to some nagging problems. After my cancer experience, I picked up viruses very easily. Of course, having a daughter in a pre-school virus factory didn't help either. I was plagued with many cases of the flu and ear infections every winter. My internist told me to do three things: First, get a flu shot every year early in the flu season. Second, to eliminate the ear infections, I should knock the water out of each ear after showers by tilting my head and whacking myself on the opposite side of the head (which fixed the ear infections but gave me headaches). Finally, he told me to wash my hands a lot and avoid shaking hands with people (which fixed the flu problems but caused me interpersonal problems). Since I started doing these three things, I never got the flu or ear infections again.

I found a great heart doctor in Pittsburgh. My heart was stable, but on the borderline. The doctor said he would put me on the transplant list if my condition ever got worse.

I could now look back and realize God had brought me through a lot. I heard a sermon once where the minister said if you want to see God's presence, look back over what He has already gotten you through.

Unfortunately, I was not doing my part. Back when I felt I would be cured of cancer, I said it would be for the glory of God. But God doesn't get much glory if you don't do anything about it. I had never given my testimony at church and had only talked to a few people about my experience. That was it. God decided to give me another medical crisis to wake me up–this time a stroke. I have the play-by-play account on the following pages:

Sunday, September 9, 1990

10 a.m.

Jennifer and Jennette got up to go to Sunday school. I did not go because I was not feeling well. I was sleeping in Jennette's bed because she had come into the "big bed" during the night and pushed me off. I went back to my room, turned on the television, and lay down in the bed to check the Reds baseball score before taking my shower. I could not find the remote control to change the channel, but I seemed to be in a partial fog. The channel was set to *Superboy*, and I remember seeing one of the girls in the show fade into a green glow. She turned into a bad woman and beat up some rough bikers. I got up and found the remote control on the dresser, but when I got back to the bed I fell down. I turned over and struggled up using my left arm because my right arm was numb. I was getting more foggy, but I could still see *Superboy*. I think I changed the channels and watched the Reds involved in a fight with the Dodgers. I think the Reds lost. I remember having a problem with incontinence, but I don't remember it happening. I lay there knowing I had to go to the bathroom and have a shower. I don't think I ever considered trying to talk.

I walked to the bathroom and tried to clean my pajamas. I got into the shower to get totally clean. I got dressed, and I think Jennifer called. I said I wasn't feeling well, and I would see her after church. I walked downstairs to clear out the washer. I went up to get my pajamas and bathrug, and I put them in the shower. I cleaned up the toilet. I couldn't deal with anything else, so I lay down on the floor in the upstairs hallway. I waited for Jennifer to find me.

12 Noon

I woke up to hear Jennifer and Jennette. I wasn't totally awake, but I think Jennifer was walking back and forth cleaning up downstairs. Jennette was taking care of me, getting pillows and (I think) stuffed animals. At that point I tried to talk to Jennifer, but I couldn't say the words. Jennifer wanted to call the doctor, but I said "NO." I wanted to ask Carolyn (Jennifer's mother) to tell me what to do, but I could not remember Carolyn's name. I remembered "Jerry" (Jennifer's father). Jennifer called Jerry and Carolyn, but they didn't know what to do.

I lay in the big bed and played with Jennette for a while. I practiced saying words to see what they sounded like. Jennette laughed at some of my words. I could say "Jennette" but it didn't sound right. I could also say "Gavin Sinclair."

I tried to get Jennifer to change my flight to Orlando because I was leaving on a business trip that night. I could say "USAir" but I could not say "American Express." I described the calendar book with the phone numbers to Jennifer. She eventually changed the flight. I fell asleep off and on, trying to remember words. I remembered needing to call "Barb" about my "posters and pages." I wanted to call "Lou," but I couldn't say "Nehmsmann" so Jennifer could look up the number (Barb Anderson and Lou Nehmsmann were two people I worked with).

Monday, September 10, 1990

1 a.m.

Around 1 a.m. on Monday morning, I still could not talk. I got frustrated with the lack of progress, so I got dressed and drove away in my car without waking up Jennifer. I went past the exit to the bridge and had to turn around. I went over the bridge and drove downtown but missed the turn to the hospital. I circled the block and arrived at Presbyterian Hospital. (I feel sorry for anyone else who was on the road that morning, given how well I was driving.) I left the car in valet parking.

I went to the emergency room and asked for the nurse. I told her I couldn't talk properly, and she asked me if I needed the Eye and Ear Hospital (?). The other nurse figured it out and took my background information. Then I did all the insurance forms. While I waited for a doctor, I called my father on the pay phone because I couldn't remember my home phone number to call my wife. I couldn't say "Jennifer" and I couldn't say "Presbyterian Hospital." My father called Jennifer after we finished talking.

approximately 3 a.m.

I talked with a doctor and two medical students. The two students talked in very clinical terms about my apparent stroke, the first indication I had of the problem. They sent me for a CT scan.

approximately 6 a.m.

I waited for the CT scan result. I talked to Jennifer on the phone, and she said Myrle and Frank were coming. Jennifer was very agitated. I talked to Barb Anderson (with a great deal of difficulty) about her plans for the Orlando trip.

I talked to a speech therapist and later to the doctor I had seen earlier. He explained the CT scan result. Meanwhile, they stuck me eight times (literally) to get blood. Then the results were wrong and they had to do it again. Where was the Sloan-Kettering blood man when I needed him?

By the time I got to my hospital room and had the exam, it was 10 a.m. Jennifer came shortly thereafter, and then Myrle and Frank came after flying that morning from Indianapolis to Pittsburgh.

1 p.m.

The doctors gave me a verbal test: count from 100 backwards by 7 (I was nowhere close); name as many animals as you can (I could only name 13 animals in 60 seconds); spell "fork"   (I could not even say "fork" and tried to spell it as s-p-o-r-k); what month is it? (I said the month was December instead of September); do you cut hair with an ax? (I said "of course.")

Throughout this experience, I was as clueless as when I didn't know what an "oncologist" was. I had no idea what a "stroke" was or what it did to you. I was totally confused during those early hours when my mind did not seem to be processing thoughts correctly.

I can give a simple layperson's definition of how a stroke is caused. A stroke occurs when a blood clot goes into the brain, temporarily cutting off blood flow to a region of the brain. If the blood is cut off for too long, some of the brain tissue dies, causing permanent damage. If the brain tissue is damaged, therapy can help reroute the impulses through the brain and hopefully minimize the problems. (I hope there are no neurosurgeons reading this simple explanation.)

Stroke victims are usually given blood thinners, such as Coumadin or even aspirin. The blood thinners don't actually "thin" the blood, but they reduce the clotting tendencies of the blood. This helps prevent any more clots from forming, but they make shaving with a dull blade an interesting experience.

My stroke was caused because my heart was not pumping very efficiently, and in some crevice of the heart, a clot formed. Somehow the clot broke free, entered my blood stream, and found its way to my brain. This is not scientific, but the day before my stroke I went to a batting cage for the first time in years. I am totally convinced it was my mighty hits of the ball that jarred the blood clot loose in my heart.

The brain does an amazing job of repairing itself. Within a week, I was back to 90% comprehension. The experience gave me empathy for a whole new class of people, this time stroke victims. You can't imagine the frustration of knowing something in your head, but not being able to communicate this thought to other people. The mother of one of my friends had a stroke shortly after me (her name was Margaret Balest). I am usually not the most sympathetic person, but I could understand the frustration in her eyes when she tried to communicate something. I think it made her feel better knowing someone else understood what she was going through.

There was a major turning point during this hospital stay that affected the rest of my life. One night, one of the elders from my church, Tim Morrison, came to visit me. In this conversation, I was finally able to put together what God had done for me through my many illnesses. Tim eventually motivated me to give my testimony at church. I typed out a copy of my testimony and gave it out to people having health problems. That four-page testimony ultimately led to this book.

You lose a lot if you don't learn anything from going through a serious illness. You lose even more if you don't tell other people how God was faithful to you.

God has put certain people in my life to share experiences. One of these people is Chuck Stauffer. I got involved with the hospital visitation ministry at church, and the visitation pastor, Bob Barrett, put me in touch with Chuck. When I met Chuck, he had been confined to bed for the past ten years. Chuck had five different back surgeries, each of which had left him worse off than before. He suffered from continuous pain and frustration from being confined to bed.

I visited with Chuck about once a week. It was a good experience for both of us. I was the only one who could really understand the pain that Chuck was going through, and seeing Chuck made me more appreciative of how God had taken me through my problems. Chuck has a wonderful wife, Margaret Stauffer, who has helped Chuck through his trials. It is hard on the person who has to live with someone going through pain. Margaret explained her feelings to me on a little tape recorder that I loaned to her.

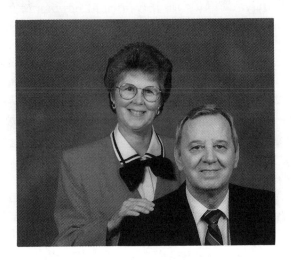

Chuck and Margaret Stauffer

From Margaret Stauffer:

I've got to tell you, Gavin, this is really difficult for me. I have trouble even talking on an answering machine, let alone this thing.

I'm going to try to give you some of my thoughts about loving someone who deals with pain. Loving someone who deals with pain constantly has been a very difficult thing. I guess my first idea when Chuck started having pain was I needed to fix it. I'm a mother, and I fix everything. You either kiss it or put a Band-Aid on it or you distract them. If that doesn't work then you find somebody who can fix it. In Chuck's situation we couldn't find anyone who could fix it. I came to the point where I felt helpless. I felt helpless because I couldn't fix it. A lot of frustration came from that.

The next thing I wanted to do was to make a deal with God. I thought, "God, if you make him better, then together we can do a lot of things for You." Chuck and I had talked about going into missions together. He had so much talent. He could sing. He had a lot of charisma. "There is so much he could do, Lord," I prayed. "Why does this have to happen to him?"

But then, after a while, I realized that number one, I couldn't fix it and number two, God doesn't need my help. Trying to do something is what was causing my frustration. When I realized that God could do this without me was when it led me to a more complete trust, a trust that realized God would do in the whole situation what was best. God knew and understood the pain that Chuck was going through. He was using the situation for His purpose. He was also using me in my role for His purpose.

I finally came to the point where I could say, "This is completely out of my control. This is where God has placed me, and this is what God wants me to do. I will do it the best way that I can." I found a sense of peace by just letting God use me.

Another thing that I found helpful was learning not to worry about tomorrow, or five years from now; not to fret about a situation getting worse, or worrying about the unknown or what was going to happen. I just tried to get along that day. I got up, and I did that day what I had to do that day. I was not so worried about tomorrow.

"Therefore, do not worry about tomorrow, for tomorrow will worry about itself. Each day has enough trouble of its own." (Matthew 6:34)

I try to look for positive things in each day, not negative. I try to appreciate the things that are good like friendly visits from wonderful people like you, calls from friends, or visiting with my grandchildren. Sunshine is wonderful for me. Just plain feeling good is a blessing.

"This is the day the LORD has made; let us rejoice and be glad in it." (Psalms 118:24)

I must say that verse to myself twenty times a day. Sometimes I have to be careful that I don't try to twist Jesus into my mold. Instead, I need to be willing to be transformed into His mold. There are some things in my life that I would like to change. If I could be a genie and rub a lamp and Jesus would do what I asked, then I think I could tell Jesus some really good things that He could do for me. I think we all could. But the reality is that true religion isn't to conform God into my image, but for me to be conformed into His image. So it's not whether God will do what I want Him to do, but the question is, "Am I going to do what God wants me to do?" When I can get this through to myself, it takes a load off my shoulders. All I have to do is what God wants me to do. All I have to do is live the life that He has given me and do it the very best that I can.

I am confident that something good comes from everything, including my stroke. Maybe it was meeting Chuck and Margaret Stauffer and learning from them. Maybe it was finally motivating me to tell my testimony to others. I may not know the answer, but I'm sure that God works these things for good.

About a year after my stroke, I got a good scare. One morning, when taking a shower, I felt a lump near my right armpit. It was about the size of a marble. My first thought, of course, was cancer.

I made an emergency request to see my internist. He said he would see me over his lunch hour. He was a part-time doctor who saw patients half the day and did research the other half. Whenever I looked for a new doctor, I always asked if they liked challenges. This scared away all but the very curious and brave doctors, and I have found some very good doctors using this technique.

My internist felt the lump and confirmed the obvious. "There is definitely a lump, but there is no way to tell if the lump is malignant or benign." He sent me to see a surgeon immediately. The surgeon felt the lump, and said he would take it out. It was a small lump, so he could do it on an out-patient basis using local anesthesia. He said to schedule the surgery with his secretary at my convenience.

The secretary was still on her lunch break, so I had to call her back that afternoon. It was the Monday before Thanksgiving. I was getting a little paranoid about this lump, and I wanted it out as soon as possible. I told the secretary I wanted the surgery the next day, Tuesday, or Wednesday at the latest. She told me that would not work, and I would have to wait until the following Monday.

If I had not been thoroughly trained in how to deal with the hospital scene, I would have said okay. I wasn't going to accept this answer, however, because I wanted the lump gone before cancer could spread through my body.

"That is unacceptable," I told her. "The surgeon said he would do it at my convenience, and I want it done tomorrow or Wednesday." One of my previous bosses taught me the power of the word "unacceptable." When you use this word, people automatically seem to want to work out a counterproposal. Saying something like "that is not good enough" seems to leave the onus upon you, and the other person doesn't seem as willing to try to come up with another solution.

"Let me talk to the surgeon," the secretary said, "and I'll get back to you." She called about five minutes later and said the surgery would be on Wednesday.

I went to the hospital on Wednesday morning. I changed into a gown, and I was put on a stretcher. The nurses shaved my armpit and sterilized the area. Then I was given some pills and a shot to numb the area. A half hour later they wheeled me into the operating room.

The doctor was there with two residents. I was totally conscious during the whole operation and talked with the doctors about what they were doing. I always found that knowing what was happening kept me more relaxed. The surgeon told me when he had removed the tumor, and I immediately asked him what it looked like. "Looks like a lump of fat," he said, "I doubt if it's malignant." The surgeon asked if I minded if one of the residents got some practice closing. I said to go ahead, happy to do anything to help get these residents trained correctly. The surgeon stayed and directed the young resident through the quick process of sewing up the four inch incision.

I went for the follow-up appointment on Friday to get the biopsy results and so the surgeon could check the incision for infection. When the surgeon came in he said, "Well, I'm very surprised."

"What do you mean," I asked tentatively.

"When I took the lump out, I felt certain the lump was malignant," he confessed. "When the pathologist said the lump was benign, I went to look at the slide myself because I couldn't believe it. But he was right. The lump was benign."

"But you told me it looked benign when you took it out," I responded.

"I know," he said, "I always tell people that so they don't worry."

There's a lesson there somewhere, but at the moment I was just glad that the lump was benign. The incision was healing fine, and I went home happy.

There seem to be two philosophies when it comes to giving a prognosis. Some doctors tell you the absolutely worst thing that can happen, figuring that you will be happy when it turns out better than expected. Others, like this surgeon, tell you not to worry regardless of how bad the situation may be. In any case, statistics and forecasts are meaningless when applied to a single person. The doctors can give you the odds of what could happen, but a 99% chance of something happening doesn't mean that's how things will turn out for you. I always liked getting feedback from the doctor, but I always remembered it is impossible to predict what would happen with certainty, and I never got too overconfident or too pessimistic.

After cancer, congestive heart failure, spinal surgery, drug addiction, stroke, and a benign tumor, this brings "Part I: My Story" of this book to a conclusion. It's amazing how God gives you the strength to endure any situation. I do not consider myself brave or courageous. Problems were thrown at me, and I responded as best I could.

The real heroes were the ones who had to suffer through this experience with me. While I was the focus of attention, it was my family and friends who prayed for me, worried about me, and took care of me. The next section of the book relates their stories.

PART II: FROM ANOTHER ANGLE

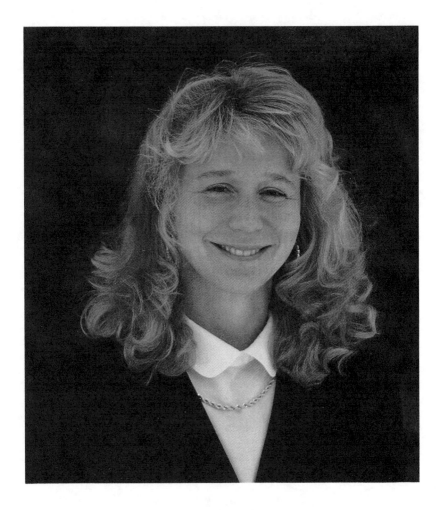

Jennifer Sinclair

Chapter 11: From My Wife

I met my wife, Jennifer Doloresco Sinclair, in freshman chemistry class at Purdue University. She later told me she thought I was a geek because I sat in the front row. Our first date was not a promising beginning. I wore a tight turtleneck to show off my muscular body. She told me I looked like a pinhead and I should change my shirt. I then took her to see the movie "Apocalypse Now" which I thought would be very romantic in a gory, Vietnam War sort of way. When she told me she didn't like it, I told her she was shallow.

From this auspicious beginning, we fell in love and got married at the end of our sophomore year. Besides being in love with her, she was also getting straight A's in chemical engineering and I needed help with my homework.

My wife is the strongest person I know. As my mother wrote earlier in this book about Jennifer, "Can you imagine having a husband in the hospital with inoperable cancer, and you in graduate school and pregnant?" Through the whole experience she rarely complained about having to care of me.

Here is what Jennifer had to say:

My mother and father told me about the real seriousness of Gavin's illness in the parking lot of Frisch's restaurant
in Cincinnati. I hyperventilated and cried a little. They helped
me calm down by reassuring me in different ways–telling me
all the things the doctors could do for Gavin and the many
different types of cancer he could have, some of which were
highly curable. We told Gavin that night after we got back to
my parent's house. My mother did most of the talking, and she
presented the situation to him pretty much as she had to me. At
that time we didn't know what kind of cancer he had, and we
were hoping it was lymphoma or something similar with a high
cure rate. I was optimistic that all would work out.

Gavin was admitted to the hospital the next day. About
a week later Dr. Morgan came into Gavin's room with the biopsy report. Gavin's parents and two of his friends were also in
the room. Dr. Morgan explained the seriousness of Gavin's
type of cancer, and that he probably only had four months to
live. After the doctor told us the diagnosis and prognosis,
Gavin's parents and friends immediately left the room with the
doctor and his nurse. I tried to talk to Gavin but he wanted to
be alone, so I left his room. When I went out into the hall,
Myrle and Frank were crying and Dr. Morgan's nurse was trying to comfort them. I couldn't take that scene. I wasn't ready
to cry like that, crying in resignation to what I believed they
saw as something inevitable. I just didn't see it that way at all,
and I was not ready to give up. I couldn't resign myself to
Gavin having four months to live when the doctors had not
even done anything for him yet. I knew that cancer treatments
succeeded with some patients and not with others, and it
seemed reasonable that Gavin could be one of the successful
cases.

I believe anything is possible with God. Many people
might say I was not in touch with reality, but the doctor's pro-
nouncement of four months to live was surely not "set in

stone" in my mind or my heart. I did not believe the doctor's words were the end of the story. For many people with cancer and their loved ones, a doctor's prognosis is seen as final and all hope is completely lost at that point. While taking into consideration that physicians are generally held in awe in our world today, and while I do have respect for them, I know firsthand through my educational experiences that advanced degrees do not guarantee great knowledge or a level of competence that is beyond question or thorough examination. As capable as they may be, physicians are not God.

A few days later Gavin went for a radiation treatment. My brother Bryan and I were in the room when they wheeled Gavin away. I recall being very happy that day thinking that the doctors were *doing* something for him. I felt that the radiation would at least stop the cancer growth and for that I was very grateful. I remember that Bryan and I prayed that day in the hospital room. We prayed not that Gavin would get well, but that God's will would be done. We prayed that Gavin, and others, would be brought closer to Christ through this experience. This was truly my deepest desire. I knew that if Gavin was right with the Lord, everything would be okay and God would take care of the rest. After I said that prayer with my brother, I had a sense of peace that somehow Gavin would be all right. He would overcome this cancer.

Gavin's hospital stay was challenging in several ways. The first that comes to mind was receiving visitors. People would come wanting to show their love and concern, and some brought gifts. When Gavin didn't feel like talking, I was unsure how to handle the situation. I didn't want Gavin to be irritated, but I also didn't want our visitors to feel as though we didn't appreciate their care or gifts. On those occasions, managing the conversation was difficult. Food gifts were especially awkward. Gavin always graciously thanked the people, but he just could not eat most of the food. When they asked later if Gavin enjoyed the food, I didn't know how to respond. In the beginning of Gavin's illness, I would lie and say he really enjoyed it. As time went on, knowing that lying was wrong, I was able to be more honest about his situation. For the most part, the other people were very understanding and appreciative of my candidness about Gavin.

When Gavin was in the hospital and at home, I tried to be a good nurse to him, although this is not one of my strong suits. I never cared much for being around sick people and germs. It's amazing how my attitude changed once Gavin was sick. Feeding Gavin, waiting on him, getting to the hospital very early to shower him as he sat on a chair (for he was too weak to stand), surely seemed like no big deal to me compared to what he was going through.

I also had to clean his trach twice a day. The tracheostomy hole opened right into his windpipe. I remember one time while I was cleaning the trach at Mom's house that Mom came to watch. She said she never thought she would see the day when I would start acting like a nurse.

I also recall my father-in-law Frank telling me one morning early in Gavin's illness how highly he thought of me for supporting Gavin. That comment from Frank meant so much to me and I kept it in my heart all during Gavin's illness. It spurred me on when I was growing weary because I knew helping Gavin was what I needed to do no matter what, regardless of how I felt emotionally or physically. Remembering this helped a lot when I was feeling selfish or depressed.

I felt sometimes that Gavin's perpetual coughing was going to drive me crazy. It was so irritating. I knew he couldn't help it, but he would cough and use tissues and they would be in tons of wads all over the floor by his bed. I got tired of picking those wads up all the time. What a stupid little thing to get to me, but it did.

In more of a general sense, sometimes I would be alone and start having a pity party for myself, thinking I was married to an old man because he acted like that. Again, I knew he couldn't help it. A few times I did let these feelings take over. One time we were visiting Bryan and Amy (my sister-in-law) at their married student's apartment in Purdue, one just like we had while at Purdue. We had just visited one of my former professors at Purdue earlier that day. Gavin had his trach at this time, we had to drag oxygen around, and he did not look very good. This professor thought very highly of me at Purdue and was a major influence leading me to attend Princeton. I felt after that visit he just didn't think the same of Gavin and me, as though before he saw us as "winners" and now as "losers." That night, when I lay in bed at Bryan and Amy's apartment after Gavin was asleep, tears streamed down my cheeks for a very long time thinking about how Gavin and I used to live in an apartment like this with so much to look forward to and now everything seemed all messed up. I believe I learned a lot that day about the true inherent worth of people's titles, degrees, notches on the ladder of success and how these things are viewed in certain people's eyes. I learned that true friends are there through everything, not just when things are going well and you are on the fast track. I was reminded that worldly success is fleeting and does not compare to the love of my husband, family and Christian friends. I also was taught more fully through this experience that real, lasting happiness and peace comes through doing the will of God, however lowly or unsuccessful in the world's eyes that may be and whether or not you feel you are being blessed by the Lord or rewarded by anyone else. I cannot say I do not forget these truths sometimes. I need many reminders, but thankfully the Lord provides them. In my profession as a college professor, I continuously struggle with the lure of worldly success, measured by other professors and researchers, rather than concentrating on pleasing God. Without Gavin's cancer experience to draw upon, I would not be as cognizant of this temptation area in my life.

During the summer of 1986, after his surgery, Gavin went into a deep depression. He stayed upstairs in bed every day, all day long. He hardly ate, which was a very serious concern to me. I was always trying to encourage him with different types of foods. He hardly talked to his parents when they came from Indianapolis. He wouldn't hold Jennette, and, worst of all, he just didn't seem to want to do anything to help himself get better. One day I couldn't take it any longer and I told him he was "useless." I know I said it out of selfish motives, and I made Gavin mad at me. As it turned out, Gavin later thought this was just what he needed to hear.

Another time, about three weeks after Jennette was born, Jennette was screaming, Gavin was sick in bed and not able to do anything, and I was trying to get my computer modem working. I needed to connect to the Princeton computer and start doing my computer modeling for my Ph.D. research at home. I couldn't get the modem working after multiple attempts and couldn't calm Jennette down. I felt like I was going to crack. I felt like I would never be able to get anything done again. Taking care of a sick husband, a baby, and trying to finish a Ph.D. seemed to be overwhelming. I wanted to give up. I cried for a long time and then decided crying wasn't going to solve any of the problems, so I started in on everything again. I knew giving up was not the answer.

What did help the most through the first year after Gavin's diagnosis were two things. First, Gavin was generally positive through most of his illness, except for his depression in the summer. He even drove me to the hospital ten days after his surgery when I was ready to deliver Jennette and stayed with me during the delivery. Second, Christian relatives and friends were a great source of support for me. In particular, Charlotte Riley, my next-door-neighbor and Lamaze coach; Joyce Bolton; and Norman and Caroline Feiss helped by taking care of Jennette during Gavin's treatments or when I had to go in for meetings at Princeton. They were always praying and always willing to help me. These two factors kept me going, along with the faith I had from the Lord.

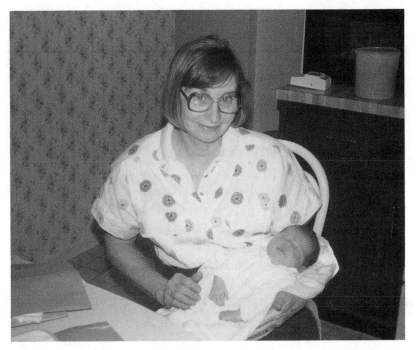

Charlotte Riley and Jennette

Although the time after Gavin's cancer diagnosis and subsequent treatments was long and difficult, the most intense fear I had was when he had his stroke. Jennette and I were at church that Sunday morning; Gavin did not go because he was not feeling well. When we got home I found Gavin lying on the hallway floor sleeping. I woke him up and he was acting strangely, coherent in some things and not in others. I thought at first he was just kidding around with me like he often does. He said he didn't know my name, yet he knew other people's names. I found his dirty pajamas in the shower. I didn't quite know what to make of the situation. He was acting *very* weird. I didn't know what to do. I called my mother, who had learned a lot by working in a doctor's office for twenty years. I considered the possibility that Gavin may have had a stroke, but he did not have the typical symptoms like numbness on one side that my mother told me about. In fact, physically he was fine. I was not sure what to do except let him rest in bed, which is what he mostly did that day. While I was asleep that night, he drove himself to the hospital. I didn't even know Gavin was gone until I got a phone call from his father in Indianapolis.

When I got to the hospital, the neurologist told me Gavin had experienced a stroke. Then he began to ask Gavin a series of questions—what was the date, what was his address and phone number, and questions involving the meaning of certain phrases like "crying over spilled milk." Gavin could not answer any of the doctor's questions. I went a little crazy. Here was my highly intelligent husband not being able to answer very simple questions virtually any adult (and most children) could answer. He was not himself mentally. My immediate reaction was that I needed to somehow convince the doctor that my husband was not stupid and that he was not acting like his normal self. I began to ramble on frantically, telling the doctor my husband was a National Merit Finalist, he had a 145 IQ, and he graduated with two degrees from Purdue University in four years. I know I behaved completely irrationally, but I was overcome with worry. To me, my husband was no longer like the husband I had known for ten years. Even when Gavin was going through all of his treatments and surgery and everything else, he was still Gavin and acted like Gavin and behaved and talked in a way that was consistent with Gavin. But suddenly this was no longer true. The doctor tried to calm me by telling me he was very sure my husband was intelligent and the fact that Gavin couldn't answer the questions was to be expected. However, in my crazed state, I just felt like the doctor was patronizing me.

Later that day the neurologist informed us that he believed Gavin had experienced a mild stroke, and he expected Gavin to have almost a complete recovery mentally. In fact, after about three weeks, Gavin was essentially back to his normal self. His only residual problems involve remembering series of numbers (never trust him if he tells you a phone number), relating a logic/puzzle correctly (for example, saying "my sister's husband's sister" would require some time on his part to get it straight in his mind), and using the wrong words or switching the order of things when talking, especially if he is tired. However, these are small things that other people do not notice during Gavin's typical daily interactions.

It is difficult to relate the relief I felt after the neurologist informed me of Gavin's prognosis following his stroke. I was more relieved than at any other time during Gavin's illness, even including the report from the surgeon immediately following Gavin's tumor removal at Sloan-Kettering. I still believe that nothing could be worse *for me* than to have Gavin, or any other loved one, be in a different mental state than their normal state. *For me*, if Gavin had to remain in bed his entire life requiring constant physical attention but yet was himself mentally and we could carry on conversations, it would be far, far better than to have him in a state in which he was fine physically but altered mentally. Praise the Lord Gavin had essentially complete recovery from his stroke.

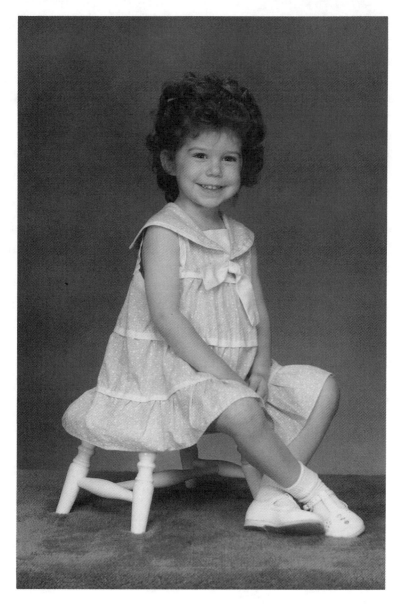

Jennette Sinclair, age three

Chapter 12: From My Daughter

My daughter, Jennette Sinclair, was the one who gave me the motivation to live. Writing that letter to my "unborn child" was the turning point. Before then I wasn't sure whether it was God's will for me to live or die. After looking at the "Dear _____," I felt it was God's will for me to live.

Jennette truly has me wrapped around her finger, and she takes advantage of it at every opportunity. She wrote this when she was ten years old:

When Dad had his cancer, he thought he would never meet me. He wrote a letter to me starting "Dear _____." But, to everyone's surprise, he did meet me.

I have to be patient with my dad. He can't play sports that well, but at least he can play them a little. I'm glad he didn't die of cancer. Often I forget that he had cancer and I get too rough with him. But once when we were fighting about the remote control he lifted me up onto his six-foot-tall dresser. I couldn't get down until he helped me. I guess he's not so sick! But he acts like he broke his leg when he stubs his toe.

Here are some great advantages of having a weak dad: Always winning in wrestling, always sitting in the front seat of the car on night trips (he loves to sleep on night trips), and no need for an alarm clock. Coughing wakes me up at 4 a.m. Here is the bad part: Hospital trips, just because of a cough. And you have to get used to looking, feeling, and hearing *very gross* stuff. It's easy to get used to. Sometimes it's pretty cool.

I don't remember my dad's cancer. Well, why should I? I wasn't even born. The only sickness that my dad had that I was alive for was his stroke. He once whispered to me after he had his stroke, "Jennette, what's your mom's name?" I was only four or five then, so I giggled and thought he was being silly. I said, "Silly, you know what Mommy's name is!"

My dad got very lucky when he had cancer. I can tell it in just three words: He didn't die. I feel lucky that my dad D.D. (didn't die).

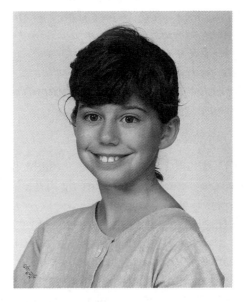

Jennette Sinclair, age ten

Chapter 13: From My Sister

My sister, Mareth Sinclair Gunstream, is everything I am not. She is three years older than me and she is a saint. I tormented her throughout our childhood, but she was always kind and polite. Mareth graduated from Wheaton College with a degree in music. After college she married Robby Gunstream. Robby is the executive director of The College Music Society, and they live in Missoula, Montana with their three children: Corbin (whom you heard about earlier in this book), Caroline, and Colin. Mareth also has a Master's degree in counseling, which she probably uses to prevent her children from tormenting each other like Uncle Gavin did to her. Here is what my sister wrote:

Looking back ten years ago, some things have faded from memory and others remain vividly.

My dad called during the Christmas holidays in 1985 to tell me the cold Gavin had was more than just a cold. He started to tell me about an upcoming biopsy. He was not speaking very coherently and then he abruptly hung up. I was befuddled, to say the least. Thankfully, Gavin called right back and said it was no big deal. He told me everything was going to be okay, and he wasn't going to die or anything. I told him I loved him and we said good-bye.

A few days later, when we learned he had cancer, I immediately flew to Indianapolis from Boulder, Colorado with my two-year-old son, Corbin.

Gavin was in the hospital in Cincinnati and we made the trip over there the first week in January. I remember feeling better just being in closer proximity to him, but I wasn't prepared for what I saw. He looked so sick and couldn't talk very well because of the tumor pressing on his vocal cords. I tried to smile and be upbeat, but when we got back to the hotel room that afternoon, I was completely exhausted, both physically and emotionally. I slept for two hours or so.

So many memories and feelings of those days crowd in. I recall going to the gift shop at the hospital and wanting to buy things for Gavin, perhaps because I felt I really couldn't do anything for him. I didn't know whether to show my fear and sorrow or to appear happy and joke about everything. I also remember trying to entertain a very active two-year-old son in the hospital. We had a game about trying to keep his toes on the line in the waiting room and not go out into the hall.

After Gavin's tracheostomy, we all took turns being in his room. I remember the strange sound the trach made and wondering if Gavin was all right. I was perspiring heavily, convinced he was going to expire then and there on my "shift."

We met wonderful people on Gavin's floor. One woman, whose husband had died of cancer two years earlier, was there with her dad. Most of the nurses were also wonderful, caring individuals. One of the nurses who worked the night shift had lost her husband to cancer. I had never met so many people affected by cancer in such a short time.

We started staying in Cincinnati on the weekends, and during the week we went back to Indianapolis. Every night in

Indianapolis after I got Corbin to bed, my parents and I would talk about the latest findings from the doctors.

After about four weeks we decided I should return home. When I got home I remember thinking how insignificant most things I did or worried about seemed. Who cares about shopping or looking at the latest things out on the market? I felt angry with the people at the mall–wondering how they could merrily go on with their lives. Didn't they know my brother had cancer and the doctors said he was going to die? I also remember (very irrationally) being mad at Gavin because he told me in that first conversation that he wasn't going to die and now they said he was.

Every night when I tucked Corbin into bed, he would pray, "Dear God, Please let the tumor shrink. In Jesus' name, Amen." It was literally the only thing I could pray for in those weeks. My life seemed consumed by radiation reports, chemo-therapy reports, and doctor reports. I felt guilty going out and having fun with my family and friends. Gavin's cancer was the first thing I thought about waking up and the last thing I thought about before going to sleep.

The months passed and in the spring I went to visit Gavin and Jennifer in New Jersey. I accompanied Gavin to Sloan-Kettering with Corbin in tow. That place in itself was an experience. I couldn't believe virtually everyone I saw had can-cer or was with someone who had cancer.

When New York drivers would pull out in front of us as we were driving to Sloan-Kettering, I wanted to yell at them, "Don't you think you could be a little more considerate? My brother has cancer, he's not feeling well, and you just cut him off."

I couldn't believe the price of parking at Sloan-Kettering. I remember thinking, "Don't you think if you had cancer you should be exempt from paying the parking bill?" Seeing all the children with cancer really broke my heart.

I marveled at how calm Jennifer was, in spite of Gavin's illness, being pregnant and finishing her doctorate. I almost wondered whether she had heard the same news that the rest of us had.

I had a friend have lunch with me during the time I thought my mother would call me with the news about Gavin's cancer surgery. I had so many friends and relatives I knew were praying for us during the entire time, and that helped tremendously. People still ask me ten years later, "How's Gavin?"

A sense of what's really important always hits home during something like this. I don't assume I will live to a certain age. I have more empathy for people with cancer and their loved ones. I am grateful that Gavin's illness helped me learn these lessons.

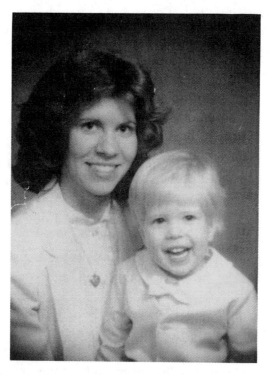

Mareth and Corbin Gunstream in the summer of 1986

Chapter 14: From My Friends

From Charlotte Harrington:

My parent's friend, Charlotte Harrington, was a very important source of strength for them throughout my illness. Charlotte actually went to high school with my sister. I barely knew her. Charlotte graduated from high school and then went to Ball State University in Muncie, Indiana for a degree in education. She is a teacher in Indianapolis. Here is what Charlotte had to say:

Ten years ago seems like an absolute lifetime. In my case, it probably is, since the person I was then is, thank you Jesus, radically different from who I am today.

I remember that Gavin's dad, Frank, had left a message on our answering machine saying that he wanted me to pray for Gavin–a mass had been found in his chest. No details. What? A mass? People die from those things!

In short order, the details became clear, partly because I am admittedly one of the nosiest friends anyone could have–at least in the detail department. I wanted to know *everything*. Everything was not good for Gavin Sinclair.

Remembrance of this period in "history" allows me to reflect on what I consider a critical issue. When Gavin was diagnosed with cancer, the prognosis included the harshest possible reality. Gavin was going to die. At this time, I was going through one of several periods where I thought I would too. Not really, but I had some real problems. I was single with some serious boyfriend problems. Anyway, Gavin's illness jolted me into a new way of thinking. What was going on in my pathetic existence *did not matter* all of a sudden. What *did* matter was that Gavin get well. Now, how was that going to happen when all signs pointed to a certain death?

The Bible says that *all things work for good for those who love God and are called according to His purpose.* Far be it for me to argue with the Bible. The following are some "good" things that resulted from something as horrible as a terminal diagnosis:

Charlotte (that's me) stopped thinking about herself for a change. She was able to recognize that her accursed singleness was a blessing for the Sinclairs, who needed someone to stay with Gavin's "Gramma" whenever the family was away for one of Gavin's procedures. I was a free person. I could do this. I wasn't encumbered by the family I so wished I had. This was for good.

I participated in prayer meetings at church. Every mention of Gavin's name, whether in a formal prayer meeting for him, or in the announcements at the beginning of the service, or in the prayer requests at choir, was met with immediate tears. Big ones. I didn't even really know Gavin. But I did know his mom and dad, and they were two of the most special people in the entire world. I loved them, and I did not want them to hurt. I really didn't know what it was like to "love God" at that time, and I certainly had never allowed Him to call me to do anything, but I did know what it was like to love

Gavin's mom and dad. *This couldn't happen to them. Gavin must get well.* Gavin *did* get well.

Reportedly, many people besides me have been affected by Gavin's story. Gavin is a Christian who is not afraid to share his testimony. Gavin was healed by a miracle from God, no less than what you read about in the Bible. Physical healing is real. Emotional healing is real.

Take everything to Him. He is there, and He listens, and all things do work together for good. Do you love Him? Have you allowed Him to call *you* according to His purpose?

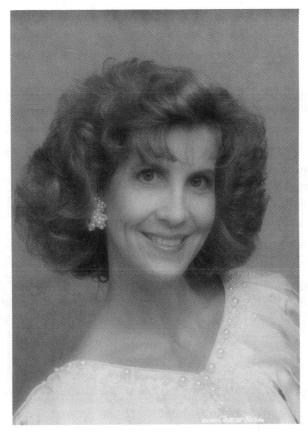

Charlotte Harrington

From Vincent Bonaddio:

Vinney was a friend of mine from Air Products, the company I worked for when I was diagnosed with cancer. Vinney and I were part of a "rat pack" composed of people in their early 20's who started working for Air Products after college. Vinney is one of those people you can always depend on, and he is always very careful to be straight and honest in all relationships.

Vinney was in the room when I received my original prognosis of four months to live (my wife and parents came in a few minutes later), so he has a unique perspective.

I am having a difficult time remembering when I met Gavin. I guess that just means it was a typical occurrence in a typical day. At the same time, I cannot say that Gavin has been a typical person in my life. I got to know him when we worked together on several projects during my first job out of university. My first exposure to his illness was in Atlantic City during a sales meeting. He had already been diagnosed with bronchitis and was taking some antibiotics. I remember distinctly that he asked me not to make him laugh because of the tremendous amount of pain that it caused. Naturally, as a good friend, I did my best to make him laugh. It was all in good fun and I certainly did not know the extent of what was about to occur.

I definitely remember the first day back from the Christmas holidays when the group was called into Larry Iceman's office, the manager of the group that Gavin and I both worked in. Larry told us about Gavin. I went numb and I really didn't know what to do.

I followed my heart and did my best to get to Cincinnati, Ohio. I made arrangements with my girlfriend Lauri (who is now my wife) to travel that weekend to visit Gavin in the hospital. I didn't know what to expect. When Gavin and I got together in Cincinnati, I had an opportunity to spend some time alone with him. We talked briefly about my future, and I asked him for his opinion about getting engaged to Lauri. He basically gave me the thumbs up. That was a very special moment for me, and it was very important that he approved of my decision because of our special friendship.

It was later that day, January 11, 1986, that Lauri and I happened to be sitting with Gavin when the doctor came in. He said he wanted to talk to Gavin, and Gavin said it was all right if we stayed. The doctor explained the rarity of Gavin's cancer to him and gave Gavin the prognosis of four months to live. I could not believe how Gavin handled the news. He used his slate (he could not talk at the time because of his trach) to ask several questions of the doctor, but he did not seem to show any response to the doctor's statement that he had four months to live. I was in shock. I did not know how to feel, but I certainly could not show any emotion because of the way Gavin was handling it. He was the one going through this, and I was the one trying to fight off my emotion. It just didn't make any sense.

Lauri and I left after a few minutes and I can remember breaking down in the elevator just shaking my head, tears in my eyes, because at that point I was unsure about the future. Gavin's prognosis was especially difficult for me because I had lost my father to ALS (Lou Gehrig's disease) three years earlier when he was only 49, and I didn't want to lose someone else close to me. I left the hospital with the feeling that Gavin was the strongest person I had ever met, and if anyone was going to defeat the illness through the proper state of mind, it would be Gavin. Ten years later, as I sit here pondering what has occurred, he has done it.

Over the past ten years, I have referenced Gavin's hardships as a guideline for how he is able to put his priorities in place. I work long hours in my job, and Gavin has always encouraged me to spend more time with my family. It wasn't until I read his manuscript that a lot of what he had been saying sunk in. He has never taken the time, only because it is completely against what he believes, to make me a part of all of his suffering. I found it very difficult to read Gavin's story because such a special person does not deserve to experience all these problems. I feel so close to everything he has been through, yet so distant because I cannot imagine what he feels.

I know that I have tremendous potential to become a better person specifically because of Gavin. I have never told him so, but I love him dearly in a way that words will never express. He has filled a part of my life I did not believe that I needed. I have done my best to communicate with God that His will be done and whatever prayers Gavin and his family may have will be granted.

Shortly after my father passed away, a friend asked me, "What did you pray for when your father was ill?" I told him I prayed my father would not suffer any longer. My friend said I should be thankful to the Lord for granting my prayer. My father was no longer suffering. So, as Gavin mentioned in his book, we all need to be careful what we wish for and at the same time, we need to understand our prayers, what they mean, and begin to deal with them with faith in our heart.

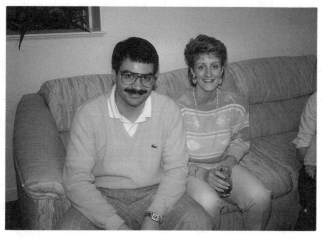

Vinney and Lauri Bonaddio

Gavin's response to Vinney's writings:

I learned some important lessons from what Vinney wrote. First, we all react differently when we hear a doctor's prognosis. My initial reaction was to be extremely calm. My wife, as she wrote earlier in her chapter, did not react emotionally. I think it's safe to say that Jennifer and I are both weird (we are, of course, both engineers, so weird is probably an occupational hazard). For most people, an emotional response is more likely and probably more healthy.

I made a mistake in not sharing more of my feelings with friends like Vinney. A good friend does not shut out other people, even in an attempt to be strong and shoulder the burdens himself. Vinney said he benefited from what I wrote, but if I had not finished the manuscript for this book, all of the gain for Vinney would have been lost. Many people learn from their experiences, but few end up writing a book about them. Sharing feelings with your friends is about the only way they can benefit from your experiences. I am not good at discussing "feelings," but I should have been more considerate and done it anyway.

Vinney said I didn't deserve what I went through. This is a natural reaction. When my father was diagnosed with prostate cancer, one of his friends called and said she was mad at God because my father had cancer. Here is what my father wrote in his journal:

Evening of June 7, 1993

A friend from our church called to say she was mad at God about my diagnosis.

We have all said wrong words when we are hurt and upset about something or someone. To have a friend diagnosed with a threatening disease can bring out thoughts from the top of our minds. This was the

121

case with my friend being mad at God. It is very hard to comprehend God's plan for our lives. We must trust Him; we must be so trusting in hard times that we become like hind's feet on a deer. When a deer's hind feet track exactly with the deer's forefeet, the deer is completely in sync.

The Sovereign God is my strength, He makes my feet like the feet of a deer, he enables me to go on the heights. (Habakkuk 3:19)

I think Vinney got to exactly the right point at the end of his writing when he said, "I have done my best to communicate with God that His will be done." When my mother had an aneurysm in early 1996, I prayed for her to get better if this was God's will, but asked for the strength to deal with the situation if God's will was for her to die. I also prayed for God to give strength and understanding to the other people close to my mother. I no longer struggle with the question of whether it is fair. I have seen God do tremendous things in "bad" situations with me and with others. My mother turned out fine, but if she would have died, I could have accepted it as part of God's plan with no feelings of anger or resentment. Learning to accept God's will has freed me from wondering about why things happen or if they're fair. Rather, I can move ahead with trust and hope in Him.

PART III: PUTTING IT ALL TOGETHER

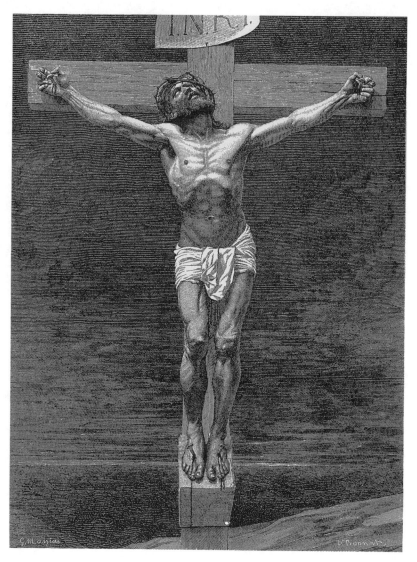

"The Christ" by Bonnat

Chapter 15: The Spiritual Lessons

Before deciding to fight the good fight against a serious illness, we need to come to grips with the following:

1. If I die, I'm going to heaven.

2. I will accept God's will.

3. All things work for good.

4. Suffering is not necessarily bad.

None of these four statements break any new theological ground. If you gave Christians a true/false test on these four statements, I think everyone's grade would be pretty good. The difference is *knowing the right answer* versus *staking your life on living them*. If you believe these four statements, you can get through any serious illness.

1. If I die, I'm going to heaven.

If you have accepted Jesus as your Savior, you can find great comfort in the promises in the Bible. If you die, you are going to heaven. Heaven is a better place than earth. There is no reason to be afraid of death if you are going to heaven. At the times when I thought I might be close to death, such as when I was in pre-op for my first surgery, I thought, "This might be the day that I go to heaven."

This book is, by necessity, a Christian book. Quite frankly, without being able to depend on the promises in the Bible, I do not know how a person can deal with a serious illness. If there is nothing more to life than what we have on this earth, there is nothing of significance. It is only a matter of time before some part of the body wears out or stops performing properly, and that's the end.

Consider my case if I had not been a Christian. I was diagnosed with cancer and told I had four months to live. Many non-Christians would simply believe the doctor. There are no miracles. There are only statistical relationships. If a *doctor*, one of the highest authority figures on this earth, says you are doomed, it probably seals your fate. Some people will turn to unconventional methods to try to extend their life, probably because they are afraid of what happens after death.

It is this fear of what happens after death that probably makes many consider religion. For many, it is not that they had previously considered religion and rejected it, although that certainly happens. Instead, I would guess that many people never bother to think much about religion because it is not a crucial issue at the time. When you are diagnosed with a serious illness and possible death, your religious faith suddenly becomes a crucial issue.

Why is it so much easier to face a serious illness if you are a Christian? First, if you truly believe the promises in the Bible, there is no reason to fear death.

> *Jesus said to her, "I am the resurrection and the life. He who believes in Me will live, even though he dies; and whoever lives and believes in Me will never die. Do you believe this?" (John 11:25-26)*

I think this is too simple for most people to accept. Even committed Christians tend to face death with trepidation. Is that because they doubt the Bible, or are they making things too complicated? Earth is not a Christian's home. There is a much better home awaiting in heaven. This is how Jesus explained it to His disciples:

> *"Do not let your hearts be troubled. Trust in God; trust also in Me. In my Father's house are many rooms; if it were not so, I would have told you. I am going there to prepare a place for you. And if I go and prepare a place for you, I will come back and take you to be with me that you also may be where I am. You know the way to the place where I am going." (John 14:1-4)*

The first step in facing a serious illness is to accept that death is not a bad option. The Bible clearly says that those people who have accepted Christ as their Savior have eternal life.

> *For God so loved the world that He gave His one and only Son, that whoever believes in Him shall not perish but have eternal life. (John 3:16)*

Most Christians know this is true in their mind. Until they have it in their heart, this promise of life after death cannot help them while dealing with a serious illness. If you are not fully confident of what happens to you after death, you need to go back and get comfortable with your eternal salvation. This is the first step in dealing with a serious illness. Paul had the right perspective:

> *For to me, to live is Christ and to die is gain. If I am to go on living in the body, this will mean fruitful labor for me. Yet what shall I choose? I do not know! I am torn between the two: I desire to depart and be with Christ, which is better by far; but it is more necessary for you that I remain in the body. (Philippians 1:21-24)*

If you are not a Christian, or if you are a Christian but are not sure you are going to heaven, this needs to be the first order of business in confronting your illness. Once you have resolved that question and know you are going to heaven if you die, then there is nothing to fear.

There is no downside for a Christian. If a Christian dies, he or she goes to heaven. Heaven is a better place than earth.

2. I will accept God's will.

Now that the alternative of dying seems better, let's consider the option of living. While we do not need to fear death, God may want you to be alive. From the verses above (Philippians 1:21-24), Paul believed that "remaining in the flesh" was more necessary than his desire to depart and be with Christ. In my case, I believed I needed to be there for my new baby. I do not think this is wrong, taken in perspective. In my case, I found great comfort in the promise that *all things work for good.* I knew that if it was God's will to take me off this world and take me to heaven, it would ultimately work for good.

A wish to continue living on this earth is not a bad emotion as long as it is based on fulfilling God's work for you on earth. If you are truly comfortable with your salvation, I do not think you can be *compromised* by an overwhelming desire to live. Before deciding to make a concerted effort to live, you should evaluate your own heart to determine that your desire is not based on being uncomfortable with death. If the answer comes back that your desire to live is based on your lack of assurance in eternal life, you need to go back to "Spiritual Lesson #1: If I die, I'm going to heaven."

What is the next step? A Christian can look to the ultimate Authority. Statistical predictions of who lives and who dies are meaningless when miracles are possible.

> *Jesus looked at them and said, "With man this is impossible, but with God all things are possible."* (Matthew 19:26)

It may be God's will that you overcome your illness. The most important thing is that you prepare yourself to accept God's will, whether that means life or death.

Through your illness, you have the opportunity to show people what faith in God means. If you decide to fight your illness, the most important motivation is to glorify God through your fight. The worst time to be a bad witness is in a struggle for your life. You are making a big mistake if you are making the struggle out of fear of death or a desire to fulfill things that are your will. Miracles are for God's glory, not yours.

God is in charge. Accept God's will, whether it means life or death.

3. All things work for good.

After you are convinced that you are going to heaven if you die and you are able to accept God's will, the next step is to convince yourself that all the misery you are going through will actually work for good. The Bible is very clear on this. If you love God and follow His will, everything will work together for good.

> *And we know that in all things God works for the good of those who love Him, who have been called according to His purpose. (Romans 8:28)*

It's sometimes hard to figure out how every miserable thing you go through could work for good, but if you believe it, you don't have to worry about it. To convince myself that all things could, in fact, work for good, I would try to imagine how what I was going through at a particular time could work for good. When I couldn't talk because of the trach, I imagined maybe God was preventing me from saying something stupid. When I got stuck with a roommate that complained about everything, I imagined maybe I was his roommate so I could be a good example. My original misdiagnosis may have worked for good, because I ended up being treated in Cincinnati with Dr. Morgan instead of the doctors at the local hospital. It's not very difficult to imagine how something can work for good in every circumstance. When I give my testimony in church, I always say that maybe my experience will bring just one person to Christ. The eternal benefits to that one person would certainly outweigh the inconveniences I have suffered.

The clauses to the "all things work for good verse" are very important. You must love God and submit to His will. This certainly includes doing things like asking forgiveness for your sins and putting Christ first in your life. I found that when

130

I could do that, the physical problems I was suffering didn't seem so bad anyway.

God is in charge. You don't need to wonder why these things are happening to you. Love God and obey His commandments, and the rest will take care of itself.

4. Suffering is not necessarily bad.

We are conditioned to think that suffering is bad. In fact, there are many verses in the Bible that say suffering is good. You will suffer. That's a given. Fighting an illness means suffering, but suffering is not necessarily bad.

> *I consider that our present sufferings are not worth comparing with the glory that will be revealed in us. (Romans 8:18)*
>
> *Consider it pure joy, my brothers, whenever you face trials of many kinds, because you know that the testing of your faith develops perseverance. (James 1:2-3)*

Besides building up character, suffering also helps you identify with Christ:

> *Dear friends, do not be surprised at the painful trial you are suffering, as though something strange were happening to you. But rejoice that you participate in the sufferings of Christ, so that you may be overjoyed when His glory is revealed. (1 Peter 4:12-13)*

I've also said the only thing worse than dying of cancer is being cured of it. Look at my record: chemotherapy, radiation, chest surgery, congestive heart failure, stroke, narcotic drugs, and spinal cord surgery. Once you are assured of eternal salvation, suffering is the main issue left. If it is God's will to leave you on this earth to suffer, you need to equip yourself to deal with this situation.

> *Not only so, but we also rejoice in our sufferings, because we know that suffering produces perseverance; perseverance, character; and character, hope. And hope does not disappoint us, because God has poured out His love into our hearts by the Holy Spirit, whom He has given us. (Romans 5:3-5)*

To help you deal with suffering, there is nothing better than Psalm 23. This is so familiar, it's easy to read through too quickly. Try reading it slowly and think about what each sentence means.

A psalm of David. The LORD is my shepherd, I shall not be in want. He makes me lie down in green pastures, He leads me beside quiet waters, He restores my soul. He guides me in paths of righteousness for His name's sake.

Even though I walk through the valley of the shadow of death, I will fear no evil, for You are with me; Your rod and Your staff, they comfort me. You prepare a table before me in the presence of my enemies. You anoint my head with oil; my cup overflows. Surely goodness and love will follow me all the days of my life, and I will dwell in the house of the LORD forever. (Psalm 23)

Anyone can react well to good things. Character is dealing with adversity. Suffering strengthens our faith.

Chapter 16: The Mental Lessons

The previous chapter listed the spiritual lessons that address our eternal state. This chapter discusses the mental lessons to help us keep our sanity while we're suffering on earth.

5. Be positive.

6. Laughter is the best medicine.

7. Be thankful for what you've got.

8. Do what you can and then move on.

The mental battle is much more important than the physical battle. If you can maintain a positive, thankful attitude despite your problems, you have won 90% of the battle.

5. Be positive.

There is no substitute for a positive attitude. If you don't make a concerted effort to be positive as often as you can, your circumstances can easily pull you down. If you sit around and feel sorry for yourself, when you are done feeling sorry for yourself things are not any better than before. Try to minimize the time being depressed and start to move forward.

I found it was easier to be positive when I was around people. That gave me the impetus to try to be a good example. When I retreated and stayed by myself, like I did after my first surgery, it led to depression. The more you can be out and around people, the more positive you can be.

I found visualization to be a positive response to my cancer treatments. Visualization gives you some sense of control and makes you think about the successful treatment of your disease. I think it's the sense of control that leads to the good results people see with using visualization. If you consider the opposite case, a feeling of letting the situation control you, the helplessness can certainly take away the fight that a person has for battling the illness.

You really need a regular dose of positive thinking to keep on track. Visiting positive friends, watching a weekly television broadcast like *The Hour of Power*, listening to tapes by positive speakers, or reading positive selections from the Bible are all ways to maintain your positive attitude.

6. Laughter is the best medicine.

You will encounter many situations during the course of a serious illness that are so frustrating and miserable, you will either need to laugh or cry. Interestingly, laughing almost always has a better physical effect. Laughing activates the immune system and releases endorphins, natural pain killers. Crying can depress the immune system and cause congestion. If you have to make the choice, laughing is better for your body than crying.

Going back to maintaining a positive attitude, laughing is usually a better mental choice as well. It's hard to be negative when you are smiling and laughing.

Of course, there are many times when you will cry. Circumstances will guarantee that. In the cases where you have a choice, try to laugh.

> *A cheerful heart is good medicine, but a crushed spirit dries up the bones. (Proverbs 17:22)*

Laughter is a proven way to improve your health, both mentally and physically.

7. Be thankful for what you've got.

It may be an overused phrase, but that probably just means it's true: Be thankful for what you've got. This entered into my thinking very early in my illness when I came up with the two questions I had to answer when facing my terminal illness: "Where do I go when I die?" and "Am I happy with what I've accomplished?" My answer to the second question was "No," largely because I was not thankful for what I had. I spent my whole life trying to work towards something better without being thankful for what I had right then.

When your illness takes away certain abilities, it is even more important to be thankful for what you have. I never appreciated taking showers very much. Then I was forced to take sponge baths for weeks so I didn't get my IVs wet. Next I couldn't take a shower because I would get my surgical incisions wet. When I finally got to the point where I could take a shower, I was very thankful. I try to stay thankful even now for being able to take a shower, and I think back to when I couldn't to remind me.

I wish I would have been thankful for things that I have now lost. I used to sing in high school, even singing in Carnegie Hall and Kennedy Center. After high school, I never sang again. I was never very thankful for the voice that God had given to me. I remember telling my sister on the way to Sloan-Kettering one day that I would start singing again if my voice allowed it. Because of the paralyzed vocal cord, I cannot sing anymore. All the years I had the ability but didn't use it were lost.

This is another good reason to visit sick people. When I visited my friend Chuck, who was confined to bed, I was very thankful I could walk. Sometimes we are not truly thankful until something is taken away. But the fact is we have plenty to be thankful for every day, even during the worst part of our illnesses.

I had a friend who was always getting upset by things at work. He would say things like "my life is ruined." One day when he said this, I asked, "Did your wife die today?" No, he answered. "Did your children die?" Again, he said no. "Do you have a terminal illness?" Not that I know of, he answered. "Well," I told him, "it seems like the most important things in your life are fine. If the top 95% of your life is fine, I don't think you should get so worked up about the little issues."

If we practice *counting up* the things that are good and stay thankful for these things, we have a totally different perspective than if we *count down* all the things we don't have.

Even during the worst times of my illness, I was still fortunate. I could see. I could hear. It was always easy to find someone worse off than me, and that helped me to be thankful. Even during the bad times, I knew there were doctors, nurses, relatives, and friends trying to make me feel better. I had much more than the people who were in concentration camps. These may seem like strange examples, but it just reinforces the point that we have plenty to be thankful for, even in the worst of times.

It is very easy to forget to be thankful for what you've got. To use the shower example again, if you've ever had IV lines in your arms that have prevented you from taking showers, you are truly appreciative of not having them for the first day. The thankfulness quickly wears off, though, until soon you forget all about it. The same could be true about almost anything. The terrible pain that kept you awake all night goes away, and soon you forget how terrible the pain used to be, and how thankful you used to be when it was gone.

I am fortunate that God reminds me to be thankful by giving me a good sharp pain at least once a day. This reminds me to be thankful that my pain is no longer chronic. I am now in the habit of starting out every evening prayer by thanking God for a relatively pain-free day. I would suggest that you identify some regular event in your life with a prayer of thankfulness. Maybe it's your morning cup of coffee or a morning shower. Maybe it's taking off your shoes at night. Whatever event you choose, it is important to thank God for what you've had that day, and it also gives some perspective that makes life look much better. Every day looks brighter if you can remember what some of the really bad days were like.

Make the most of each day and stay appreciative.

8. Do what you can and then move on.

The first questions that many ask when they learn of their illness are "Why me? What did I do? This is not fair." To the non-Christian, these are valid questions. To the Christian, are these the right questions?

First, we probably won't know "why" until we get to heaven. Was God punishing us? Maybe. Was He using this illness to test our faith? Maybe. Did He give us this illness so that we can glorify Him by our response? Maybe.

There are a number of possibilities, none of which is helpful to dwell on. God has His reasons, and we are not going to know them right now regardless of how much we think about it. Our job is to respond properly.

There are some things that are helpful to dwell on. There are other things that have no answer. To make the best use of your mental strength, you need to make critical decisions about what will be the focus of your efforts. In most cases, trying to figure out why you are sick is a waste of time. You are probably not going to know. Focus on positive efforts to deal with your illness.

Anyone can react well to good things. That does not take faith, courage, or character. Instead of trying to figure out why this happened to you, focus your mental energy on how you will have the courage to react well to a "bad" thing. Focus your mental energy on how to be a good example to other people. Focus your energy on actions that move you toward the goal of fighting your illness.

My father had a very hard time during my illness. During one of his visits, I told him, "Man is too simple to contemplate one thing too long." I hope I did not unintentionally steal that from someone else. It sounded to me as if it should have been said by some famous philosopher before me. My point was not to overwork a thought. Most of these life or death issues are actually very simple. If you die, you go to heaven. If you believe this, it is very simple. If you overwork it, you will never find the answer. If you come up with a question that cannot be answered simply, you are probably not going to figure out the answer. Moreover, it is probably not an answer that would help you in the task at hand anyway. Even if you were to learn "Why me?" that would not help you with your battle against the illness.

Don't torture yourself with questions you cannot answer. First, set things right with God. Then, forget about the unanswerable questions and move on.

Chapter 17: The Physical Lessons

Ultimately we need to translate our good attitude into action. In this chapter I have listed the critical physical lessons:

9. Set goals.

10. Never give up.

11. Be in charge of your medical care.

You may be frustrated because you can't do everything you used to be able to do. Set realistic goals and keep pushing forward, never giving up.

9. Set goals.

The way to surmount any problem is to take it one step at a time. *Inch by inch, everything's a cinch!* Goal setting is crucial when recovering from an illness.

Theoretically, if you make progress every day toward a goal, eventually you will get there. This should be your attitude when you are recovering from an illness. Sometimes it is overwhelming at the beginning. It's natural to think about what you used to be able to do, and what you can't do now. The best approach is to set a goal on what you can achieve with whatever new limitations you have, and start taking small steps toward that goal. The first step is the hardest step. Once you get started on the path to recovery, you can make it.

Most illnesses leave you depleted of energy. Other illnesses can leave you without certain abilities, like the loss of the use of an arm. It can be frustrating not being able to do what you used to do. The first thing to do is to face the new reality. Consider the case of handicapped children. Many have been handicapped since birth, which can be an advantage in some ways, because they never knew what they were missing. If you see children running a race at the Special Olympics, their reaction after winning a race is not unlike the reaction of a sprinter running the 100 meter dash at the Olympics. The kids in the Special Olympics have adjusted to their reality. Their definition of success is different from the definition of the world-class Olympic sprinters. When you are faced with new limitations, you need to adjust your reality in the same way. You need to set goals that are meaningful in relation to your new reality.

Set goals. Take a small, positive step toward your recovery every day.

10. Never give up.

Probably the most notable aspect of successful people is that they never give up. You have probably heard the stories: successful authors got 300 rejections before their first story was accepted, Thomas Edison tried thousands of different ideas for the light bulb before he finally came up with a design that worked, and so on. It is even more important to persevere when you are facing a serious illness.

> *He gives strength to the weary and increases the power of the weak. Even youths grow tired and weary, and young men stumble and fall; but those who hope in the LORD will renew their strength. They will soar on wings like eagles; they will run and not grow weary, they will walk and not be faint. (Isaiah 40:29-31)*

Setbacks are part of any serious illness. In the process of fixing one problem, another problem is created. It is one struggle after another. Hopefully the problems get smaller, but somewhere in the string of problems a larger one can jump up. This is the easiest time to throw in the towel. But from what I've seen, once a person gives up, it's very difficult to get back on track.

I tried to look at every problem as a separate battle. I never thought of my congestive heart failure, my spinal surgery, or stroke as a continuing series of problems. I saw them each as separate battles, and approached each problem with a new sense of perspective. By taking each problem as a manageable little piece, I did not get as discouraged or feel the desire to give up.

From the beginning, you need to tell yourself that giving up is not an option. You need to persevere at all costs. Giving up negates all the hard work you have put into your recovery, both in terms of the medical treatments as well as the example you have provided to others.

> *I can do everything through Him who gives me strength. (Philippians 4:13)*

There will be many times when you feel like giving up. Resist the temptation! The only way to win the fight is to *never give up*.

11. Be in charge of your medical care.

The biggest mistake most people make is to think their doctor is in charge of their medical care. After all, the doctor is the expert. Doctors are trained in medicine and they deal with medical problems every day. The natural reaction is to let the doctors tell you what to do.

But doctors are only specialists hired by you to do a job. You, or more likely your insurance company, are paying them. Doctors will be an important part of your recovery, but certainly not the only factor. Nurses, friends, relatives, and most importantly, *you* play an equal or greater role than the doctors. You must get to the point where *you are in charge*.

Doctors, by their nature, are very sure of themselves and, for the most part, very intelligent. They are also very businesslike and *probably have never gone through what you are going through*. Most people are intimidated by their doctor. If they call the doctor with a problem, they wait until the doctor calls back. If the doctor says to have a test done, they do it without questioning. This attitude is changing in the days of "second opinions," but most people still have a great reluctance to challenge doctors or to "bother" them with your problems. If you are not this type of person, that's great. If you are, consider the following: Many doctors are simply too busy to return all of their phone calls. Some doctors have told me they judge the importance of a problem by how many times the patient calls. So don't hesitate to call repeatedly. But don't call if it's not important. Doctors also know which patients complain too much. When in doubt, you should err on the side of calling too often and being too forceful.

Many doctors have an efficient nurse or assistant that can handle most problems. If you are having problems reaching a doctor, ask if there is someone else you can call with your questions. Often this person has the doctor's "ear" and will make sure the doctor is aware of your problem. In many cases, the doctor's assistant can answer your question directly.

Given the vast amount of information that a doctor must deal with, it is not surprising that some things get lost. You should expect to spend a lot of your time tracking down test results and making appointments with specialists. If the doctor tells you he or she will take care of these details, don't believe it. Give the doctor a chance, because many doctors are good with this or have staff members that take care of it. In many cases, however, you could wait forever. If the doctor misses dates for getting you information or making appointments, take the initiative and make the call yourself.

Remember, your care is the most important thing to you and is always foremost in your mind. Doctors have to deal with many patients, all with important needs. If the doctor cannot put your needs first every time, that does not suggest he or she cares any less. It probably just means the doctor is very busy. Most doctors do not mind if you take it upon yourself to track down some loose ends, and it is certainly more productive and reassuring to you than simply waiting by the phone.

If your doctor is offended because you ask questions or get a second opinion, you have the wrong doctor. Most good doctors naturally think they are pursuing the best possible course for your care. Most good doctors also recognize that there are different alternatives. You should never hesitate to ask tough questions or ask for another opinion.

I have learned that most doctors operate based on pattern recognition. If the doctor has seen your problem before, he probably knows what to do. If he has not seen your problem before, he will make an educated guess. The greatest benefit I found from consulting several doctors about a problem was their different backgrounds. Once I had a chronic cough. First I went to an allergist, who suggested allergy shots. Next I went to an ENT, who suggested I had a reflux condition (stomach acid backing up into the throat). Next I went to a pulmonologist, who suggested I had a lung infection. Each prescribed a course of action based on what they had seen in the past. All were very good doctors. But only one of them was right (the pulmonologist). Unless you are willing to see many doctors, you may never find the one with the correct pattern recognition.

I have many other examples of this. When dealing with my pain, I tried at least fifteen or twenty different courses of action. When I had high fevers after my vocal cord operation, it took three attempts before finding the real problem.

The best way to improve your odds of finding the solution is to go to the biggest hospital you can. If you have cancer, go to one of the comprehensive cancer centers (like Sloan-Kettering). There is a much greater chance that they have seen other people with your problem. They are also more familiar with side effects, complications, and related factors. A common event that I see all the time is when a person with a problem goes to their small local hospital, receives a diagnosis, and proceeds immediately with the treatments at that hospital. At minimum, if you get the initial diagnosis from a local hospital, you should then go for consultation at the biggest hospital you can find. If they agree with the original diagnosis, you can decide whether to have the treatments at the local hospital or the bigger hospital.

Local hospitals certainly have some advantages over large medical centers. Their staff is more personalized and usually has more concern for your mental state and attitude. They are often located closer to friends and relatives, so people may visit you more often. And for many treatments, the care at a local hospital can be as good as a large hospital. For example, once a chemotherapy regimen is defined, it can be given almost anywhere. On the other hand, for surgery I would definitely go to a large hospital if your circumstances allow it. The support services at a large hospital tend to be better as well. Something as simple as taking blood samples was a big problem for me at my local hospital. At Sloan-Kettering, they had people who took blood samples all day long, and they are very good at it.

You should also be aware of the biases most doctors have. Family doctors spend most of their time treating people who do not have serious problems. In my case, the family doctor in New Jersey continued to think I had bronchitis, because in his experience that's what almost all the people who presented my symptoms had. On the other extreme, medical students spend a lot of their time dealing with people who have serious problems. They are more likely to think your problem is more serious than it may be.

I was very fortunate to have Dr. Morgan involved in my care. In almost all cases, he had the right balance of what to get excited about and what to ignore. In one of my series of follow-up appointments, he compared my previous x-ray with the current x-ray. I noticed that the previous x-ray had a red circle on it. "What's the red circle," I asked.

"Oh," said Dr. Morgan, "the radiologist thought that was a tumor, but it's gone in the new x-ray."

"Why didn't you tell me last time," I asked.

"I didn't think it was anything," he said. "These radiologists always are circling things. If it was anything, we would have caught it on the next appointment. I didn't want you to get worried about nothing."

It is very hard to find a doctor with that balance. Usually they report everything or report nothing. You should measure which tendency your doctor has and then ask questions and follow-up accordingly.

Dr. Morgan was also good at coordinating the many doctors involved in my care. Some doctors are not very good team players, and they don't go out of their way to make sure all the doctors are aware of your condition. Dr. Morgan networked well with the other doctors. For example, my radiation pneumonitis was diagnosed because Dr. Morgan talked to my radiation oncologist. If your doctor does not network well, you need to contact the other doctors involved in your care directly.

Hospital stays sometimes provide good assertiveness training opportunities. One time, during my stay for the spinal surgery, the nurse gave me an unfamiliar pill. "What's this?" I asked her.

"It must be the generic form of the drug you are taking," she told me. "Go ahead and take it."

"No," I said. "I want to make sure I am taking the right thing."

She grumbled and left to call the pharmacy. She came back about a half hour later with my familiar pill. "They sent me the wrong pill," the nurse explained. Who knows what the other pill really was.

Taking blood was a particular problem for me. Even under the best circumstances, it often takes two or three sticks to get blood out of me. There was one technician at the hospital in Pittsburgh who did not like to do multiple sticks. Instead, she would stick me with the needle, and then maneuver the needle around *inside my arm* until she hit a vein. I even told her I didn't mind if she stuck me again, but she said that was not how she did things. The third time she came to torture me, I told her I wanted someone else to draw my blood. She was understandably offended, and she said I was the first one to ever make this request. She left and 15 minutes later a resident came by. He said there was no one else available to draw blood unless he did it, and he warned me that he didn't draw blood very often. I told him that I would rather have him do it. With the pressure on (and the dragon lady watching), he got blood the first time.

Don't be a passive observer. Take control of your medical care. It's your money and your life.

Chapter 18: The Family Lessons

I think an illness is much harder on the loved ones of the patient than the patient. The patient can take a very active role in recovery. The loved ones want to help, but there is not much they can do. I did not do very well on these lessons during my illnesses, but after reading what other people have written for this book, I think these are the right things to do:

12. Reassure your family.

13. Ask for prayers and support.

14. Visit people having medical problems.

Try to remember your loved ones are going through a difficult time also. Do what you can to help them.

12. Reassure your family.

I did not do a good job of reassuring my family, and it was not until I read what they had written to put together this book that I realized what I should have done.

The common theme in what my family wrote was they wanted to do more for me, but they felt helpless. They felt there was nothing they could do.

I think it would have been helpful if I would have told them, "I know you feel like there is nothing you can do, but I just appreciate you being here and supporting me with your prayers." I think that would have taken the pressure off of them, because they would know they were doing everything they could.

Your relatives and friends may feel helpless during your illness. Assure them that you appreciate their love, concern, and prayers.

13. Ask for prayers and support.

Prayer is a powerful thing. I think I was on at least five prayer chains and countless prayer lists. There are countless books on prayer, but let me just include one simple story here. The pastor at Casas Adobes Baptist Church in Tucson, Roger Barrier, gave a sermon where he said two things must be true to have prayer answered in the way that you request. First, you must ask for it. Second, it must be God's will. Ultimately God is going to decide the outcome, but we are expected to ask.

There is also a pretty clear Biblical directive to anoint the sick. I never thought of doing that, because I had always gone to churches that did not emphasize anointing. As I have learned more about the Biblical basis for healing, I think it is something that everyone should consider.

> *Is any one of you sick? He should call the elders of the church to pray over him and anoint him with oil in the name of the Lord. And the prayer offered in faith will make the sick person well; the Lord will raise him up. If he has sinned, he will be forgiven. Therefore confess your sins to each other and pray for each other so that you may be healed. The prayer of a righteous man is powerful and effective. (James 5:14-16)*

Your relatives and friends can offer you prayer and support. Ask for their help. It will be good for you and good for them.

14. Visit people having medical problems.

A good way that I remained thankful was to visit people who were sick. I also strongly believe that God didn't put me through all these medical problems for nothing. I think He wanted me to be a good example for others going through their own medical problems.

One of my favorite people in the hospital was Sister Bonnie Steinlage, a Franciscan Sister of the Poor. I was in a Roman Catholic hospital, and Sister Bonnie visited me the first night I was there. I had seen her earlier on the hospital video channel (broadcasting from the hospital chapel), and it was fun meeting a television star in person.

Sister Bonnie was not your typical nun. In fact, she was pretty wild. We had a lot of fun in the hospital. Sister Bonnie went on to become a nun hairdresser, and now she runs a hair salon for homeless people. She's become quite famous, and I've seen her on *CNN* and in *People Magazine*.

Because Sister Bonnie was there at my time of need, she made a big impact on my life. If Christians want to find the people who are suffering and searching for answers to the big questions, it seems that a hospital is a great place.

Praise be to the God and Father of our Lord Jesus Christ, the Father of compassion and the God of all comfort, Who comforts us in all our troubles, so that we can comfort those in any trouble with the comfort we ourselves have received from God.
(2 Corinthians 1:3-4)

Visiting sick people helps you remain thankful, and you can provide inspiration and help to them.

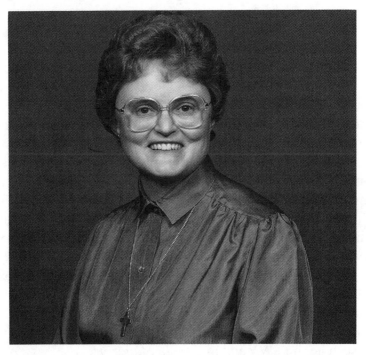

Sister Bonnie Steinlage, a Franciscan Sister of the Poor

SUMMARY

The Spiritual Lessons

1. *If I die, I'm going to heaven.* There is no downside for a Christian. If a Christian dies, he or she goes to heaven. Heaven is a better place than earth.

2. *I will accept God's will.* God is in charge. Accept God's will, whether it means life or death.

3. *All things work for good.* God is in charge. You don't need to wonder why these things are happening to you. Love God and obey His commandments, and the rest will take care of itself.

4. *Suffering is not necessarily bad.* Anyone can react well to good things. Character is dealing with adversity. Suffering strengthens our faith.

The Mental Lessons

5. *Be positive.* Nothing will defeat you faster than a negative attitude. You absolutely must be positive, whether you feel like it or not. People will be watching you to see how you react. Show them the strength from being a Christian.

6. *Laughter is the best medicine.* Laughter is a proven way to improve your health, both mentally and physically.

7. *Be thankful for what you've got.* You might be bad off, but it could be worse. Appreciate what you do have. Don't dwell on what you don't have.

8. *Do what you can and then move on.* Don't torture yourself with questions you can never answer. First, set things right with God. Then, forget about the unanswerable questions and move on.

SUMMARY

The Physical Lessons

9. *Set goals.* Take a small, positive step toward your recovery every day.

10. *Never Give Up.* There will be many times when you feel like giving up. Resist the temptation! The only way to win the fight is to *never give up.*

11. *Be in charge of your medical care.* Don't be a passive observer. Take control of your medical care. It's your money and your life.

The Family Lessons

12. *Reassure your family.* Your relatives and friends may feel helpless during your illness. Assure them that you appreciate their love, concern, and prayers.

13. *Ask for prayers and support.* Your relatives and friends can offer you prayer and support. Ask for their help. It will be good for you and good for them.

14. *Visit people having medical problems.* Visiting sick people helps you remain thankful, and you can provide inspiration and help to them.

Concluding Comments

In the introduction to this book, I made the incredible statement that I was glad I had gone through all these medical problems. How can that be true?

Before I was diagnosed with cancer at the age of 24, I was on a very dangerous course. Essentially, I did not know what was important. I knew my job was important. I knew that money was important. My new house with its green grass was important, especially if the grass was very green. Somewhere lower on the list were my wife and my God.

Thanks to one large tumor in my chest, I started to learn what was important. And I was fortunate to learn before I really made a mess out of my life.

It's true I had some difficult years. But from those difficult years, I learned to be *content*. I learned I had to put God first, my family second, and everything else third. My years of difficulty were well worth it.

Life can be as happy as you make it. If you derive your happiness from God and your family, there is no limitation on your happiness. You are not dependent on money or health for happiness. Happiness can all come from within.

> *Trust in the LORD and do good; dwell in the land and enjoy safe pasture. Delight yourself in the LORD and He will give you the desires of your heart. Commit your way to the LORD; trust in Him and He will do this: He will make your right-eousness shine like the dawn, the justice of your cause like the noonday sun. (Psalms 37:3-6)*

My spiritual and mental health are now in pretty good shape, which is 99% of the battle. I still have some physical limitations, but I can deal with them. I can't play football or baseball. My golf score has gone up 20 strokes. But it's not the end of the world. I will survive.

At the end of the first section of the book, I was in Pittsburgh. My job was going well and Jennifer was doing well as an Associate Professor at Carnegie Mellon University. I even finished my Ph.D. at Carnegie Mellon while working full time.

I was still having problems with pain. Nothing like before, but I was still taking Naprosyn (a pain medication) twice a day. I was also having problems with lung infections. Since the remaining lobe of my left lung was paralyzed in place, it was prone to infection because it never moved to keep things circulating (another medical description that will make doctors cringe). The winters in Pittsburgh aggravated my condition.

Jennifer and I decided to look for opportunities in a better climate. As it turned out, the University of Arizona had an opening for a chemical engineering professor, and we decided to make the move to Tucson. My company gave me permission to do my current job out of Tucson, which was not a problem since almost everything I did was by telephone, electronic mail, or required a trip somewhere anyway.

Once I got to Arizona, the difference was incredible. I had found my promised land. My pain was gone (no more Naprosyn), and the lung infections cleared up. One of the factors leading to my better health in Tucson was warm, dry weather. The second factor seemed to be less variation in the atmospheric pressure. Whenever a storm front was coming through Pittsburgh (which is about every day in Pittsburgh), the atmospheric pressure would drop and I would get pain in my chest. Doctors are probably *not* cringing at this statement, because I have read this phenomenon is true. The last, and possibly most important, factor leading to my improvement in Tucson was I got much more exercise. The weather is so beautiful in Tucson, I would go out for walks or to play golf. My activity level increased substantially.

We were also blessed with a new baby soon after we moved to Arizona. Derek Reagan Sinclair was born on May 22, 1996. I think that brings you up to date.

The one thing I hope is that this book can bring some sense of perspective to others. Perspective is what people really need. Perspective about what is important, perspective of oneself, and perspective about God.

I learned through my experiences. Above all, I realized the Bible has all the answers that you need. When you are a committed Christian, you have nothing to fear. During the heat of the battle, confusing as it is, strive to keep Jesus Christ as your center, and you cannot go wrong.

> *I have fought the good fight, I have finished the race, I have kept the faith.   (2 Timothy 4:7)*

Appendix: Hospital Visitation

These are notes from a one-day training program for hospital visitation volunteers that Pastor Robert Barrett gave in 1994 at North Park Church (Wexford, PA).

The need for people to visit sick people is greater today than ever before. This is the result of many trends. First, the days of personal care from doctors (such as house calls, if anyone can remember those) are over. Institutional, high-tech medicine is largely becoming the standard. Second, extended family situations are becoming the exception rather than the rule. To have three generations even in the same state is becoming less and less common. Third, the role of neighbors is becoming less important. Most neighbors no longer share a common factory, a common church, or even common friends. Finally, churches are becoming larger and impersonal. Someone needs to fill this void.

Moreover, the time when people most need other people is when they are facing an extended illness or death. This is the time they really start asking themselves, "What is the meaning of my life? Where am I going after I die?" This is the best time to be available as a good Christian witness.

The first thing to understand is that you don't need any special skills to visit sick people. You are not expected to have all the answers. You are not supposed to give special theological insights. The fact that you are there, that you are concerned, and that you know that Jesus is the purpose for life is all that's required. If you sit there and say nothing, that can still be very important to the patient.

There are a few things to keep in mind when you visit people. As you will see, these are pretty simple and should not discourage anyone from visiting people. The cardinal rule is *don't talk too much, don't stay too long.* Most people feel pressure to give a very good performance when they visit someone. This pressure usually has the opposite effect. Go, show your concern, let the person talk as much as he or she wants, and then get out of there. It is better to make the visit too short than too long.

Second, don't feel you need to make any promises. You are under no obligation to come back again, to help by mowing the lawn, or anything else. If you are the type to feel overly obligated when you make a visit, you will be less likely to visit other people again. Once again, good intentions lead to the opposite effect than what is desired. You can visit a person and have no obligation to do anything. *Don't promise to do something and not do it.* It is much better not to promise anything.

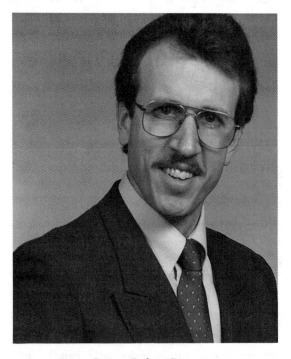

Pastor Robert Barrett

Another Story

One of the objectives of The Positive Press *is to make personal experience stories available that can be helpful to other people going through cancer or another serious illness. One of Jennifer Sinclair's graduate students, Christine Hrenya, agreed to write about her experiences when her mother was diagnosed with cancer. This story reinforces many of the points discussed in "All Things Work for Good," especially the importance of getting a second opinion and not automatically accepting a doctor's prognosis.*

The Positive Press *would like to hear how cancer or another serious illness has touched your life. If you have a story that could be helpful to others, please send it in. If there is sufficient interest,* The Positive Press *will publish an anthology of these stories.*

Late one evening, my father called to tell me that my mother was scheduled for a routine exploratory operation in hopes of determining the cause of an excess fluid buildup in her abdomen. She had already gone through the list of non-intrusive diagnostic tests, including an ultrasound and CT scan, none of which revealed the source of her ailment. I had some obligations at school the next day, so I decided to drive from Pittsburgh to Cleveland after my last meeting, which would get me to the hospital at about the same time that the operation would be ending. Going into this surgery, our family was under the impression that the possibility of cancer had already been eliminated since no tumor masses had shown up on any of the previous tests. I was about to learn just how tricky this disease could be.

When I arrived at our local hospital, my father and my sister Cheryl were waiting for me in the lobby. I knew immediately from their expressions that the news could not be good. My mother's general practitioner (GP), whose practice was located at that same hospital, had informed them that my mother did indeed have cancer and was expected to live only six to eight months. I was utterly devastated. Mom was only 60 years old. I had so much yet that I wanted to share with her. I would be graduating the following spring with my Ph.D. My husband (then fiancé) and I had been engaged for only a month. My sister had two great children, ages six months and four years. My father had taken early retirement only a few years earlier. This could not be happening to us. The three of us sat in the hospital chapel for nearly an hour and cried. Then we realized that we needed to pull ourselves together and return to my mother's room. It should have come to me as no surprise that Mom was handling the situation better than the rest of us. Though still a bit groggy from the operation, she attempted to reassure us that nothing was set in stone, and that she would fight this battle with everything she had. At this point, she was the only rational one among us. The rest of us were focusing on the doctor's prediction: less than a year left to live.

The remainder of that weekend is pretty much a blur. Mom came home from the hospital, and though we tried to be upbeat, there was definitely a somber feeling in the air. She had an appointment on Monday morning with an oncologist who was recommended to us by the GP. The GP told us that this oncologist would not only make certain my mother remained comfortable throughout the course of the disease, but also that this doctor was very good at relating to patients. I returned to school late Sunday evening, with the promise that my parents would call me immediately following the appointment on the next day.

Needless to say, trying to get work done on Monday proved quite difficult. I had an appointment with Jennifer early that day. Although I knew I would not be able to sustain a conversation on my thesis research, I was hoping that she would be able to give me some insight on how to deal with the recent news. As it turned out, she did much more than that; she was able to knock some sense into me! She told me that Gavin was originally given less than a year to live, but that she refused to believe this number from day one. As is well known, cancer is far from a well-understood disease, making it essentially impossible to predict how long any one person has to live. Jennifer also encouraged me to take charge of the situation, rather than letting the GP at the local hospital dictate our course of action. In particular, two issues needed to be addressed. First, it needed to be made certain that the diagnosis of the specific type of cancer my mother had was accurate. Next, we had to be confident that the oncologist's treatment plan was the most appropriate for that type of cancer. In other words, trust in the oncologist's expertise was essential.

Of course, this plan of action made perfect sense, and I was somewhat ashamed that I had not figured it out for myself. After all, I had spent nine years studying chemical engineering, and in that time I had been trained to research problems and think them through logically. Yet I had still taken the GP's words to be the absolute truth. To this day, I am still angered by the GP's handling of the situation. This "grim reaper" approach to the prognosis initially (and unnecessarily) stripped us of all hope that my mother might survive. And it was this hope that was essential for us not only to fight the battle ahead, but perhaps more importantly, to enjoy the time we had together, regardless of how long a period that might be. (I do not mean to imply that the GP should not have been forthcoming concerning the seriousness of the disease. However, I do strongly believe that the finality of the statement that someone only has a certain number of months to live is totally inappropriate.)

After my meeting with Jennifer, I immediately phoned my parents. To my surprise, my father sounded elated. He and my mother had just returned from the oncologist's office, and the doctor told them that my mother's chances of surviving the cancer were good! I asked my father if he knew the reason for the huge difference between this prognosis and the one the GP had given only three days earlier. He said that he was not quite sure, but that he and my mother were extremely pleased with the current prognosis, as well as with the oncologist. I also asked if they had planned to get a second opinion, but my father did not think it was necessary since they were happy with the doctor. Although I did not mention it on the phone, the latter comment did not sit well with me. It appeared as if their choice of oncologist was based purely on a more favorable prognosis rather than the expertise of the oncologist. In addition, what harm could a second opinion do? If the two oncologists agreed on diagnosis and treatment, we could stay with the current doctor. If they disagreed, we would need to gather more information and perhaps seek an additional opinion. But at least we would avoid the potential mistake of staying with a doctor who may not be the best suited to treat my mother's cancer. With this in mind, I had hoped that my parents' decision not to get a second opinion was a rash one that was subject to change. I decided to drive home that night and talk to them about it. When I arrived, they were still overjoyed at the day's turn of events. Mom was understandably tired and decided to retire for the evening. I was a bit apprehensive about telling my father what I was thinking. It is not that he is by any means unreasonable; it is just that I felt so strongly about getting a second opinion, and I would be crushed if he did not agree. As it turned out, he agreed that it was a no-lose situation. Of course, we ran the idea past my mother in the morning, and she wholeheartedly agreed with the plan of attack. In fact, she jokingly added, "All those years of college are finally paying off!"

The big challenge now was finding a doctor considered an expert who we could seek for a second opinion. My mother said that she would even be willing to travel to Sloan-Kettering (the cancer center highly recommended by Jennifer), if that would be best. The first task was confirming the diagnosis. The original biopsy suggested it was a signet ring adenocarcinoma. My mother's case was unusual in the sense that only "seedlings" of cancer were present. These seedlings were not the primary source of cancer, and the primary source was not known for certain since no large tumor mass was present (such masses would have shown up on the CT scan). However, based on the type of cancer, it was most likely that the primary source was either the ovaries or the stomach.

This information gave way to another dilemma: should we seek the opinion of an oncologist who specialized in ovarian cancer or stomach cancer or both? We did not feel comfortable making this decision with the information at hand, so I decided to call Sloan-Kettering in hopes that I might be able to get someone on the phone who could give us some insight. Fortunately, Sloan-Kettering has an 800 number set up for such inquiries. The people that I talked to were extremely resourceful, and we used this service several times. We learned that the inability to identify the primary source of cancer only occurs in about 10% of the cases. It was also explained that the only way to treat such cases was through chemotherapy, since radiation therapy is aimed at a tumor mass, which my mother did not have. In addition, they confirmed that signet ring adenocarcinoma was most often linked to ovarian or stomach cancer. But perhaps most importantly, they were able to guide us to an expert second opinion. In particular, when I first explained the dilemma of whom to seek for a second opinion, I told the staff member that we were willing to make a trip to New York. She said that the trip may not be necessary and asked where we were located. After spending a few moments searching the database, she told me that we were in luck. A highly regarded doctor who had practiced for several years at Sloan-Kettering was now the head of oncology at Cleveland Clinic, a very prestigious research hospital which was practically in our backyard. And his specialty just happened to be ovarian cancer. The search was over. We phoned immediately for an appointment.

The oncologist at the Cleveland Clinic was able to see us the following day. Based on the results of the biopsy (which were verified by a pathologist at the Cleveland Clinic) and my mother's condition leading into the surgery, he believed that the chances that the primary source of the cancer was the stomach were higher than those of the ovaries. However, because the type of chemotherapy used to treat ovarian cancer has a much higher success rate than the type of chemotherapy used to treat stomach cancer, he believed the best course of action was to first treat my mother for ovarian cancer. If she did not respond to these chemicals, a switch would then be made to the chemotherapy used to treat stomach cancer.

So what, if any, were the differences in opinion between the oncologist from the Cleveland Clinic and the oncologist that was recommended by the GP? Both had agreed on the diagnosis and the potential sources of the cancer. However, they disagreed on the plan of treatment. Unlike the oncologist from the Cleveland Clinic, the first oncologist who my mother saw recommended a more general chemotherapy plan which was not specific to any one type of cancer. The motivation here was instead of trying to hit one type of cancer hard, try to cover both bases, but with less brute force, so to speak. The logic behind both proposed treatments made sense; it was just a matter of different philosophies. Nonetheless, we all agreed that the oncologist from the Cleveland Clinic appeared to be the better choice. Not only did he have outstanding credentials, but he was also associated with a reputable research-oriented hospital, which most likely had the best possible resources available.

After these few days of research and decision-making, we all felt considerably more in control of the situation than we had earlier in the week. In addition, we were confident that my mother's chances of beating the cancer were good. Ironically, at about this time, my mother's GP called to see how we were doing. When I explained what we had learned and of our decision, the GP replied, "I admire your effort, but you do know there is no cure for cancer, don't you?" I could not believe what I was hearing! Granted, there is no universal cure for cancer, but total remission is not unheard of. In fact, according to a brochure published by the American Cancer Society, currently about 50% of all people diagnosed with cancer are predicted to be in total remission after receiving treatment. And for those survivors, total remission is nearly as good as a cure. Needless to say, this GP was not on my top ten list of favorite people.

My mother started chemotherapy the following week. My father, my sister, and I all went along for support. This was also the time when we learned some more specific information on the side effects of this particular chemotherapy. Although the side effects cannot be predicted exactly (two similar people can have different reactions to the same chemotherapy), some generalizations can be made. For instance, it was almost certain that my mother would lose her hair (she joked about going from gray to blond with the aid of a wig), while nausea was not expected to be a problem. These predictions were pretty much on target, and, all in all, my mother's experience with chemotherapy was not nearly as terrible as we had expected. (The side effects of chemotherapy have been greatly reduced between the time of Gavin's treatment and that of my mother's. I don't mean to rub it in, Gavin!)

During the weeks of chemotherapy treatments, not much could be done except to wait. My husband-to-be and I decided that it was an opportune time to get our wedding plans underway. Since we were located in two different cities (Minneapolis and Pittsburgh) and the wedding would be in yet another city (Cleveland), my mother's help turned out to be invaluable. But even more importantly, it was an activity which she enjoyed, and it helped to keep our minds off the cancer.

Throughout this whole experience, my mother never lost sight of humor. There was one friend of my mother's in particular who would come to visit her on a regular basis and tell her stories of other people she knew who were suffering from cancer. This was the last thing my mother wanted to hear. So my mom would tell her that she was tired and then go to bed. And then she would get back up as soon as this friend left! We soon coined a phrase for such stories, "Aunt Tilly stories," because they were told so frequently and by so many different people that we could not keep track of all the Aunt Tillies.

By the end of the chemotherapy, which lasted several months, it was apparent that my mother had responded to the treatments. In particular, the cancerous fluid was no longer collecting in her abdomen as it had done previously. Mom had gained back much of her energy, and the whole family felt a great sense of relief.

My mother never went into complete remission, how-ever, and later she developed serious problems battling a cough. Excess fluid again began to appear in her abdomen. She received a different type of chemotherapy, but her condition continued to worsen. A few days before Christmas 1995, the oncologist told us that the cancer had progressed too far, and that nothing further could be done. Undoubtedly, this was the single most difficult period throughout the whole ordeal. Up to this point, we made sure we had a fighting chance.

My mother passed away a few weeks after New Year's. I miss her dearly, but I will never forget all of the wonderful times we shared. And I would not be content if we had ap-proached her disease any differently. I am confident that we did everything in our power to beat the cancer, and all the rest of the while we enjoyed our time together.

Further Reading

Anderson, Greg, *The Cancer Conqueror*, Andrews and McMeel, Kansas City, 1990.

Bigley, Christine Blazer, *Cancer: A Christian's Guide to Coping and Caring*, Beacon Hill Press of Kansas City, 1994.

Bloch, Richard and Annette, *Cancer...there's hope*, R.A. Bloch Cancer Foundation, Inc., Kansas City, 1982.

Bombeck, Erma, *I Want to Grow Hair, I Want to Grow Up, I Want to Go to Boise*, Harper and Row, New York, 1989.

Cousins, Norman, *Anatomy of An Illness as Perceived by the Patient*, Bantam Books, New York, 1979.

DeCamp, Harry S., *One Man's Healing from Cancer*, Fleming H. Revell, Old Tappan, New Jersey, 1983.

Dravecky, Dave, *Comeback*, Harper Collins, New York, 1990.

Dravecky, Dave, *When You Can't Come Back*, Harper Collins, New York, 1993.

Frähm, Anne E. and Frähm, David J., *A Cancer Battle Plan*, Piñon Press, Colorado Springs, 1992.

Frähm, David J. and Anne E., *Reclaiming Your Health*, Piñon Press, Colorado Springs, 1995.

Fintel, William A. and McDermott, Gerald R., *A Medical and Spiritual Guide to Living with Cancer*, Word Publishing, Dallas, 1993.

Hill, Albert Fay; Hamilton, Paul K.; and Ringer, Lynn, *I'm a Patient, Too*, Nick Lyons Books, New York, 1986.

Larsen, Bruce, *There's a Lot More to Health than Not Being Sick*, The Cathedral Press, 1991.

Packo, John E., *Coping with Cancer: Twelve Creative Choices*, Christian Publications, Camp Hill, Pennsylvania, 1991.

Schuller, Carol, *In the Shadow of His Wings*, Jove Books, New York, 1986.

Schuller, Robert H., *Tough Times Never Last, But Tough People Do*, Inspirational Press, New York, 1983.

Siegel, Bernie S., *Love, Medicine, and Miracles*, Harper Collins, New York, 1986.

Simonton, O. Carl; Simonton-Matthews, Stephanie; and Creighton, James L.; *Getting Well Again*, Bantam Books, New York, 1978.

Sproul, R.C., *Surprised By Suffering*, Tyndale House, Wheaton, IL, 1988.

Stanley, Charles, *How to Handle Adversity*, Thomas Nelson Publishers, Nashville, 1989.

Index

A

A Cancer Battle Plan, 62
Acupuncture, 38
Adriamycin, 27
Air Products, 118
Allergist, 144
ALS (Lou Gehrig's disease), 119
Amputees, 46
Anatomy of an Illness, 24
Anderson, Barbara, 88, 89
Anesthesiologist, 78
Anoint, 132, 148, 149
Antibiotics, 13, 59, 118
Antihistamine, 23
Anti-nausea, 21, 81
Apocalypse Now, 99
Aspirin, 90
Atlantic City, 118

B

Balest, Margaret, 90
Ball State University, 115
Barnes, Dr., 38, 40, 41, 55
Barrett, Robert, 3, 91, 157, 158
Barrier, Roger, 148
Basketball, 68
Benign, 94, 96
Benign tumor, 8, 96
Bethlehem, 8, 69
Bible, 60, 116, 117, 126, 127, 130,
    131, 134, 155
Biopsy, 15, 16, 17, 95, 100, 111,
    163, 164
Blood, 38, 46, 59, 60, 72, 78, 79, 89,
    90, 145, 146
Bolton, Joyce, 104
Bombeck, Erma, 47
Bonaddio, Lauri, 7, 118, 119, 120

Bonaddio, Vinney, 3, 7, 43, 118,
    120, 121, 122
Bone scan, 9, 65
Boulder, Colorado, 23, 112
Brain, 59, 60, 89, 90
Bronchitis, 8, 13, 17, 118, 145
Bronchoscopy, 60, 64

C

Calories, 62
Capoten, 73
Cardiac catheterization, 73
Cardiologist, 36
Carnegie Hall, 16, 136
Carnegie Mellon University, 154
Casas Adobes Baptist Church, 148
Character, 131, 132, 138, 151
Chemical engineering, 99, 154, 161
Chemotherapy, 8, 9, 16, 19, 20, 21,
    27, 29, 33, 36, 37, 38, 46, 53, 57,
    60, 61, 63, 65, 72, 132, 144, 163,
    164, 165, 166
Chest bone (sternum), 41, 47
Christ, 23, 101, 127, 128, 130, 131,
    150, 155
Christian, 18, 26, 43, 103, 104, 117,
    126, 127, 128, 129, 137, 151, 155
Chronic pain, 75, 76, 82, 83, 85
Church, 43, 44, 53, 54, 86, 87, 90,
    91, 105, 116, 121, 130, 148, 149,
    157, 175
Cisplatin, 27
Cleveland Clinic, 16, 17, 163, 164
Clot, 89, 90
CNN, 149
College Music Society, 111
Compazine, 81
Computer modeling, 104
Concentration camps, 136
Congestive heart failure, 8, 9, 71, 96,
    132, 141

Cough, 41, 46, 51, 67, 102, 110, 144, 166
Coumadin, 90
Cousins, Norman, 24
Cramps, 80
Crocker, John, 53
Crystal Cathedral, 43
CT scan, 9, 23, 59, 72, 73, 88, 89, 159, 163

D

Davey, John, 7, 18
Death, 9, 10, 15, 17, 18, 24, 26, 31, 52, 54, 61, 116, 126, 127, 128, 129, 132, 138, 151, 157
Depression, 104, 134
Diaphragm, 41
Diet, 27, 32, 62
Digoxin, 73
DiLorenzo, Becky, 7
Diuretics, 73
Doloresco, Amy, 7, 103
Doloresco, Bryan, 7, 101, 103
Doloresco, Carolyn, 7, 87
Doloresco, Jerry, 51, 87
Drainage tubes, 41

E

Edison, Thomas, 140
Endorphins, 24, 134
ENT, 144
Erdis, Marjorie, 7, 51
Erdis, Maureen, 7, 51
Eye and Ear Hospital, 88

F

Faith Missionary Church, 45, 53
Feiss, Caroline, 104
Feiss, Norman, 24, 43, 104
Fever, 8, 57, 60, 80

Flemington, 8, 35, 54, 55, 63, 65, 69, 79
Flu, 85
Forgiveness, 32, 130
Frähm, Anne and David, 62
Franciscan Sister of the Poor, 149
Frisch's, 100

G

Gannon, Dr., 40
Getting Well Again, 23
Gift shop, 112
Goals, 42, 139, 140, 152
Golf, 16, 53, 154, 155
Graduate school, 16, 54, 99
Gunstream, Caroline, 104, 111
Gunstream, Colin, 111
Gunstream, Corbin, 52, 111, 112, 113, 114
Gunstream, Mareth, 3, 7, 25, 52, 111, 114
Gunstream, Robby, 7, 111

H

Happiness, 103, 153
Harrington, Charlotte, 3, 115, 117
Healing, 117, 148
Heart, 18, 20, 29, 36, 37, 41, 46, 54, 55, 72, 73, 74, 75, 86, 90, 101, 102, 107, 113, 118, 120, 128, 129, 135, 154
Heart attack, 36
Heaven, 18, 125, 126, 127, 128, 129, 130, 137, 138, 151
Hedonists, 83
Holy Spirit, 132
Hrenya, Christine, 3, 7, 159

I

I Want to Grow Hair, I Want to Grow Up, I Want to Go to Boise, 47
Iceman, Larry, 118
Immune system, 24, 32, 134
Inch by inch, 42, 139
Incisions, 41, 80
Indianapolis, 14, 16, 17, 54, 71, 79, 104, 112, 115
Infection, 64, 95, 154
Inflammation, 59
Insurance, 37, 58, 88, 142
Intensive Care Unit, 78, 79
Internist, 85, 94

J

Jesus, 22, 23, 32, 65, 93, 113, 115, 126, 127, 129, 150, 155, 157
Job, 31, 43

K

Kennedy Center, 16, 136

L

Lafayette College, 69
Lamaze, 49, 104
Larson, Bruce, 43
Lasix, 73
Laughter, 24, 133, 134, 135, 151
Lead vest, 50, 63
Lehigh University, 69
Long John Silver's, 62
Lord, 92, 93, 101, 103, 104, 107, 120, 132, 141, 149, 150, 154
Lorenzo's Oil, 55
Lung, 13, 38, 41, 46, 55, 58, 60, 68, 144, 154, 155

Lymphoma, 14, 15, 100
Lytle, Diana, 7

M

Malaria, 67
Malignant, 52, 94, 95, 96
Malignant fibrous hystiocytoma, 16, 52
Mandino, Og, 43
Marcus Welby, MD, 14
Masters golf tournament, 38
Medical Center, 14, 40
Melanoma, 44
Methylene diphenyl isocyanate, 13
Milk, 62, 106
Modem, 104
Morgan, Dr., 15, 16, 19, 20, 23, 27, 52, 53, 59, 60, 61, 65, 72, 100, 130, 145
Morphine, 75, 78
Morrison, Tim, 7, 90
Motor nerves, 77
MRI, 9, 73, 74
MUGA scan, 9, 71, 72, 73

N

Naprosyn, 154, 155
Narcotic drugs, 8, 68, 75, 77, 80, 81, 82, 83, 132
Nausea, 19, 21, 68, 72, 80, 81, 165
Nazis, 81
Necrotic, 41
Nehmsmann, Lou, 88, 119
Nerve block, 77
Nerves, 41, 77, 83
Nestles Crunch Bars, 62
Neurologist, 106
Nicklaus, Jack, 38, 39
Nutrition, 62

O

Oncologist, 15, 19, 21, 35, 36, 37, 89, 146, 160, 161, 163, 164, 166
Operation, 20, 25, 38, 41, 60, 68, 76, 77, 78, 95, 144, 159, 160

P

Pain, 26, 34, 38, 46, 63, 64, 68, 69, 71, 74, 75, 76, 77, 78, 79, 80, 81, 82, 83, 85, 91, 92, 118, 134, 137, 144, 154, 155
Paralyzed, 41, 136, 154
Parking, 88, 100, 113
Pathologist, 96, 164
Pathology, 41
Paul, 18, 31, 128
Peale, Norman Vincent, 43
People Magazine, 149
Percocet, 83
Perspective, 34, 42, 61, 67, 118, 128, 137, 155
Physical therapy, 9, 68, 75, 82
Pills, 64, 78, 79, 80, 81, 95
Pittsburgh, 8, 81, 86, 89, 154, 155, 159, 165
Pneumonia, 57, 64
Possibility Thinker's Creed, 43
Prayer, 31, 44, 45, 51, 53, 54, 92, 96, 101, 116, 120, 122, 137, 148, 149, 152
Prednisone, 27
Pregnant, 9, 14, 29, 35, 49, 50, 54, 99, 114
Presbyterian Hospital, 88
Princeton, 14, 16, 50, 54, 69, 103, 104
Prisoner of war, 34
Prostate cancer, 55
Providence Hospital, 15, 52
Pulmonologist, 144
Purdue University, 99, 103, 106
Puritans, 83

R

Radiation, 8, 9, 10, 16, 19, 20, 21, 22, 27, 38, 45, 52, 54, 59, 72, 73, 75, 101, 113, 146
Radioactive seeds, 41, 47, 50, 55
Reassure, 147, 148, 152, 160
Recovery room, 40, 46
Red meat, 33, 62
Reflux condition, 144
Religion, 26, 93, 126
Resident, 36, 37, 95
Richards, Dr., 14, 71
Riley, Charlotte, 14, 50, 104, 105
Riley, George, 14

S

Sarcoma, 16, 52
Schuller, Robert, 42, 43
Seizures, 57
Sensory nerves, 77
Septum, 58
Setbacks, 141
Siegel, Bernie, 43
Sin, 32, 50
Sinclair, Derek, 155
Sinclair, Frank, 3, 7, 45, 51, 54, 55, 63, 65, 66, 78, 79, 89, 100, 102, 115
Sinclair, Jennette, 3, 8, 50, 55, 56, 57, 60, 63, 64, 65, 76, 86, 87, 104, 105, 108, 109, 110
Sinclair, Jennifer, 3, 7, 14, 17, 27, 29, 36, 38, 45, 49, 50, 51, 52, 53, 54, 55, 60, 65, 68, 69, 76, 78, 81, 86, 87, 88, 89, 98, 99, 113, 114, 121, 154, 159, 160, 161, 162
Sinclair, Myrle, 3, 7, 45, 51, 66, 89, 100
Slate, 24, 25, 41, 119

Sloan-Kettering, 8, 29, 33, 35, 36, 38, 40, 43, 49, 54, 55, 57, 58, 59, 63, 64, 85, 89, 113, 136, 145, 162, 163
Special Olympics, 140
Speech therapy, 9
Sperm, 69
Spinal cord, 77, 83
Spinal cord surgery, 8, 9, 75, 79, 96, 132, 141, 146
Staph infection, 64
Stauffer, Chuck, 91, 92, 94, 136
Stauffer, Margaret, 3, 7, 91, 92, 94
Steinlage, Sister Bonnie, 149, 150
Steroids, 27, 60
Stortz, Ed, 78
Stress, 18, 32, 33, 36, 37, 81, 85
Stroke, 8, 9, 86, 88, 89, 90, 94, 96, 105, 106, 107, 110, 132, 141
Suffering, 34, 50, 120, 125, 131, 132, 133, 150, 151, 165
Supplements, 62
Surgeon, 19, 20, 37, 38, 41, 46, 54, 58, 78, 94, 95, 96, 107
Surgery, 8, 9, 10, 19, 20, 37, 38, 40, 41, 42, 44, 46, 47, 50, 54, 55, 57, 59, 63, 75, 77, 78, 79, 80, 83, 85, 94, 95, 103, 104, 106, 126, 132, 144, 159, 164
Sympathy pains, 49

T

Teflon injection, 8, 41, 57, 59, 63
TENS unit, 68, 75
Testimony, 90, 94, 117
The Hour of Power, 42, 134
There's a Lot More to Health than Not Being Sick, 43
Thymoma, 52
Toluene diisocyanate, 13, 27
Tracheostomy, 9, 20, 22, 24, 25, 28, 45, 102, 103, 112, 119, 130

Transplant, 86
Tucson, 8, 148, 154, 155, 175, 176
Tumor, 8, 15, 16, 17, 19, 20, 21, 22, 23, 25, 27, 29, 38, 40, 41, 51, 52, 54, 55, 59, 61, 76, 95, 96, 107, 112, 113, 145, 153, 159, 163

U

University of Arizona, 154
Update lady, 55

V

Visualization, 23, 134
Vocal cord, 8, 9, 41, 57, 59, 112, 132, 136, 144
Volunteer, 44, 78

W

Weight Watchers, 27
Wheaton College, 111
Wires, 41, 47
Withdrawal, 80, 81

X

X-ray, 14, 15, 17, 23, 27, 36, 37, 45, 47, 51, 54, 61, 65, 69, 76, 78, 145

Y

Yang, 32
Yeast infection, 64
Yin, 32

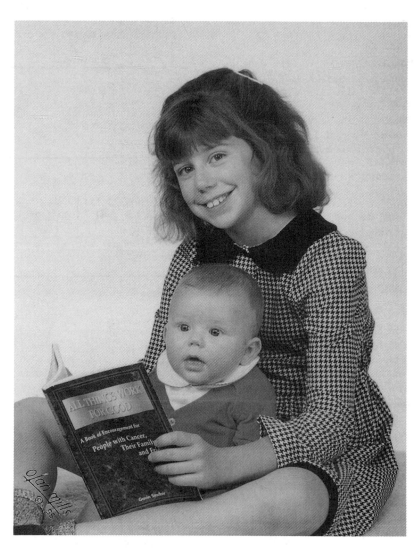

Jennette and Derek

The author would appreciate any comments about this book. You can send these comments to:

Gavin Sinclair
c/o The Positive Press
P.O. Box 32668
Tucson, AZ 85751-2668

If you found this book helpful, please ask your pastor or priest to mention the book in a church bulletin or newsletter. You might also loan a copy of the book to your hospital chaplain.

Special bulk purchases can be arranged for churches and hospitals. Contact *The Positive Press* at the address above for more information.

Order Form

I would like to order additional copies of *All Things Work for Good*. Please send to the following addresses:

Name: _____

Address: _____

City: _____ State: _____ Zip: _____

Name: _____

Address: _____

City: _____ State: _____ Zip: _____

Name: _____

Address: _____

City: _____ State: _____ Zip: _____

Please enclose a check for the following amount:

Number of copies _____ at $9.95 each $_____
              ($13.50 Canadian)

Tax (Arizona only), $0.70 per book $_____

Shipping and Handling, any quantity $ 3.00

                Total Enclosed $_____

Mail order to:

The Positive Press
P.O. Box 32668
Tucson, AZ 85751-2668

All books can be returned for a full refund if you are not satisfied.